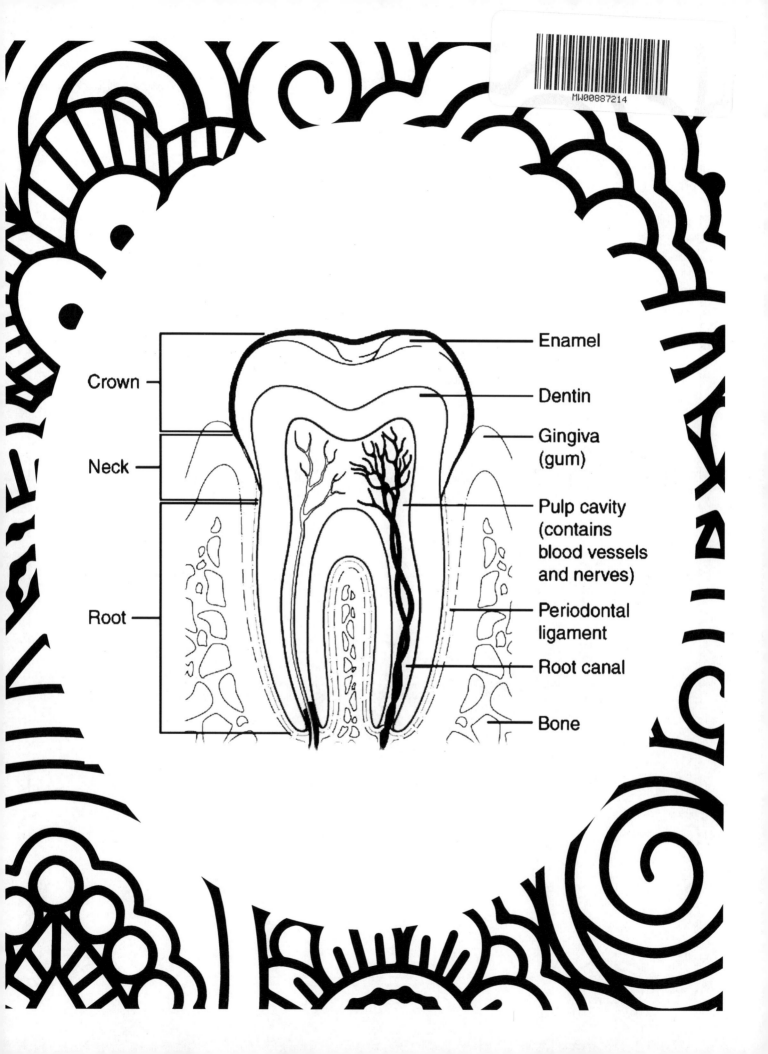

Crown

Neck

Root

Enamel

Dentin

Gingiva
(gum)

Pulp cavity
(contains
blood vessels
and nerves)

Periodontal
ligament

Root canal

Bone

This Book Belongs To

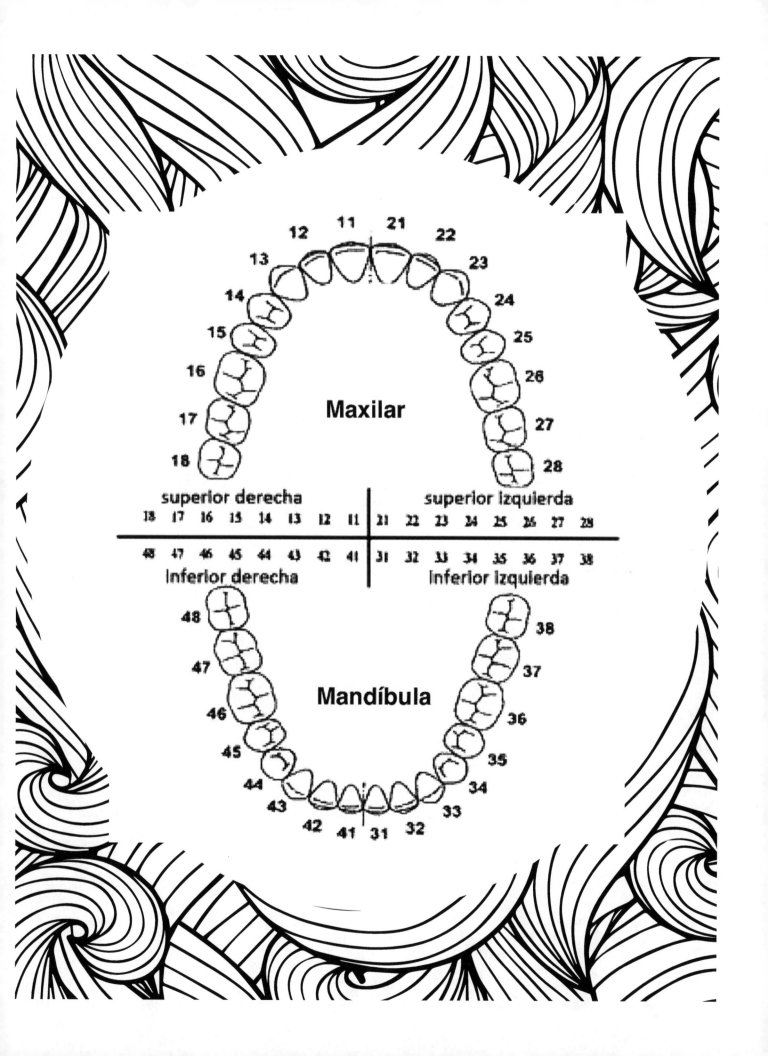

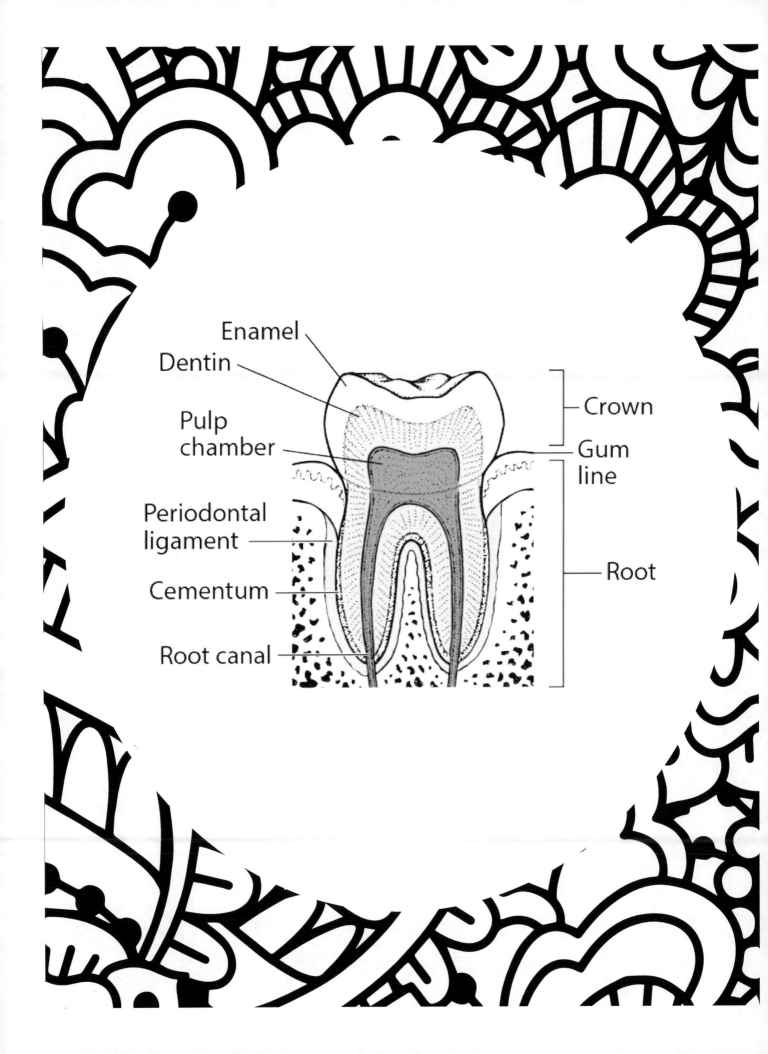

Enamel

Dentin

Pulp
chamber

Periodontal
ligament

Cementum

Root canal

Crown

Gum
line

Root

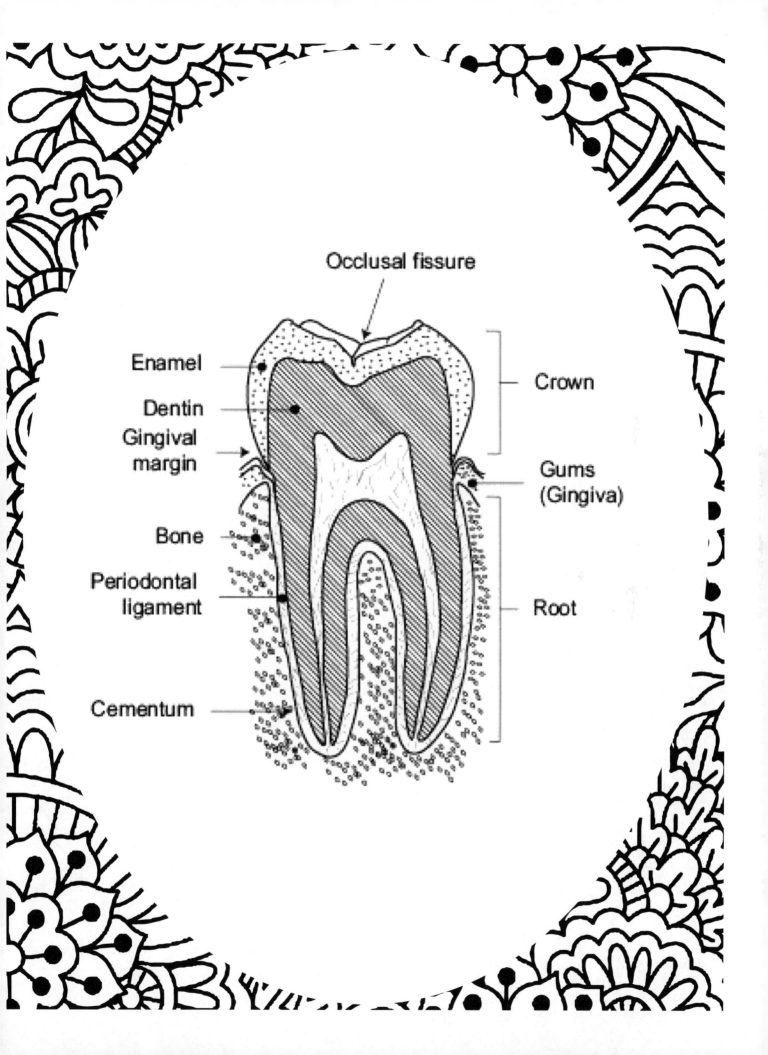

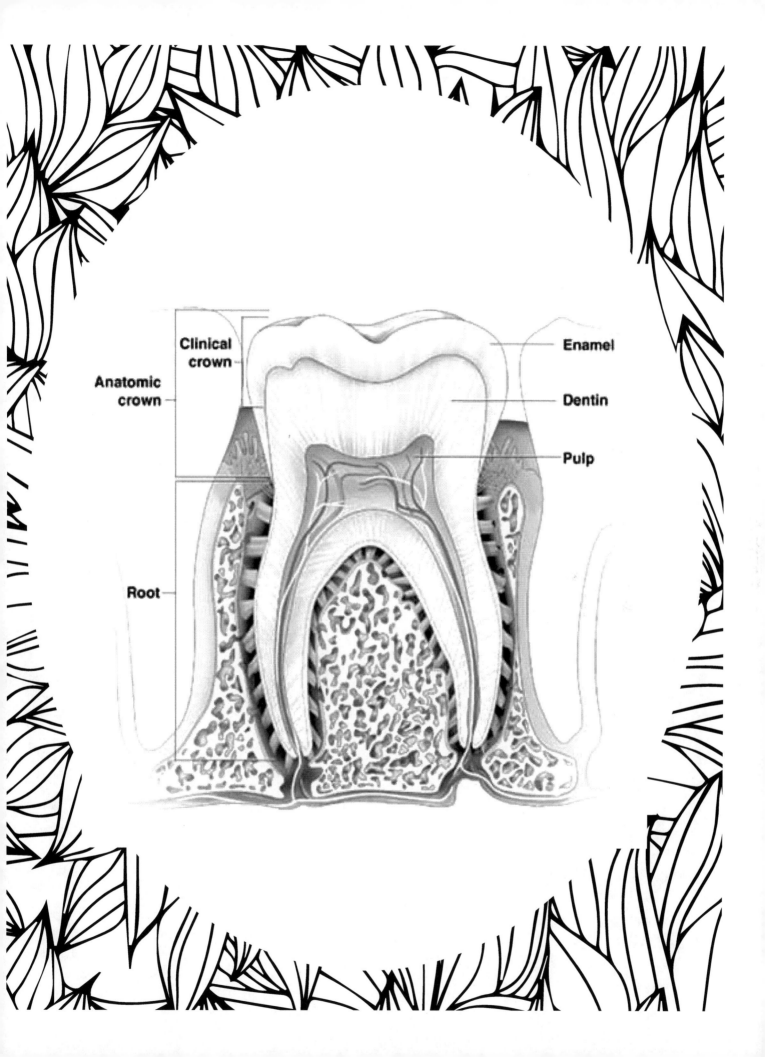

Clinical crown

Anatomic crown

Root

Enamel

Dentin

Pulp

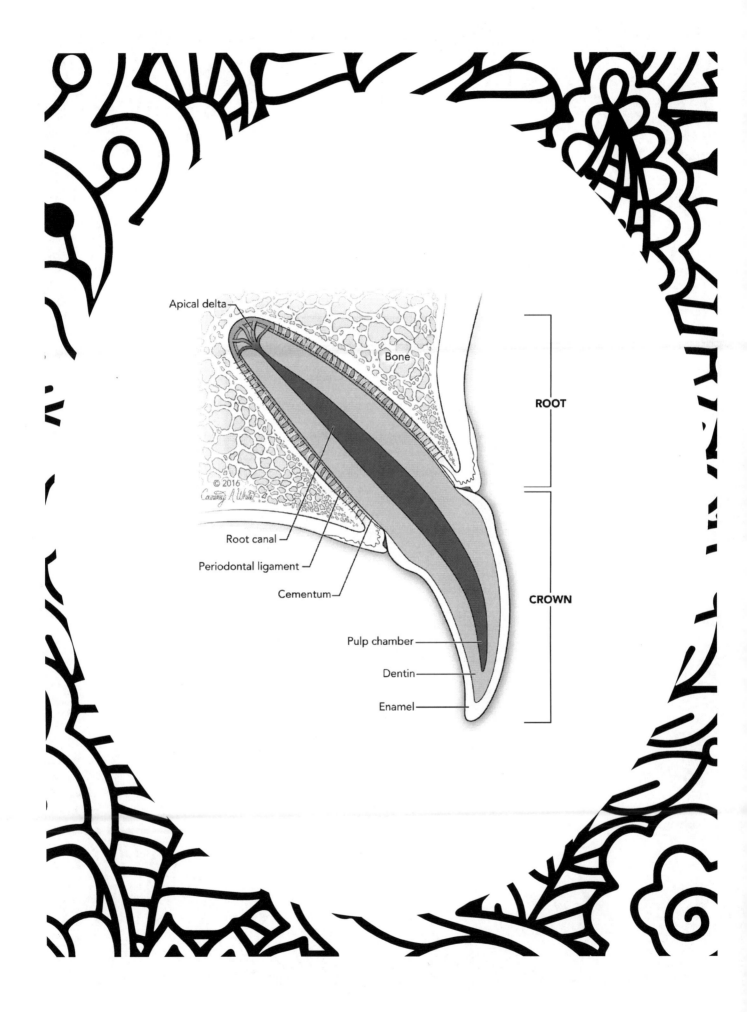

Apical delta

Bone

ROOT

© 2016
Courtney A. White

Root canal

Periodontal ligament

Cementum

CROWN

Pulp chamber

Dentin

Enamel

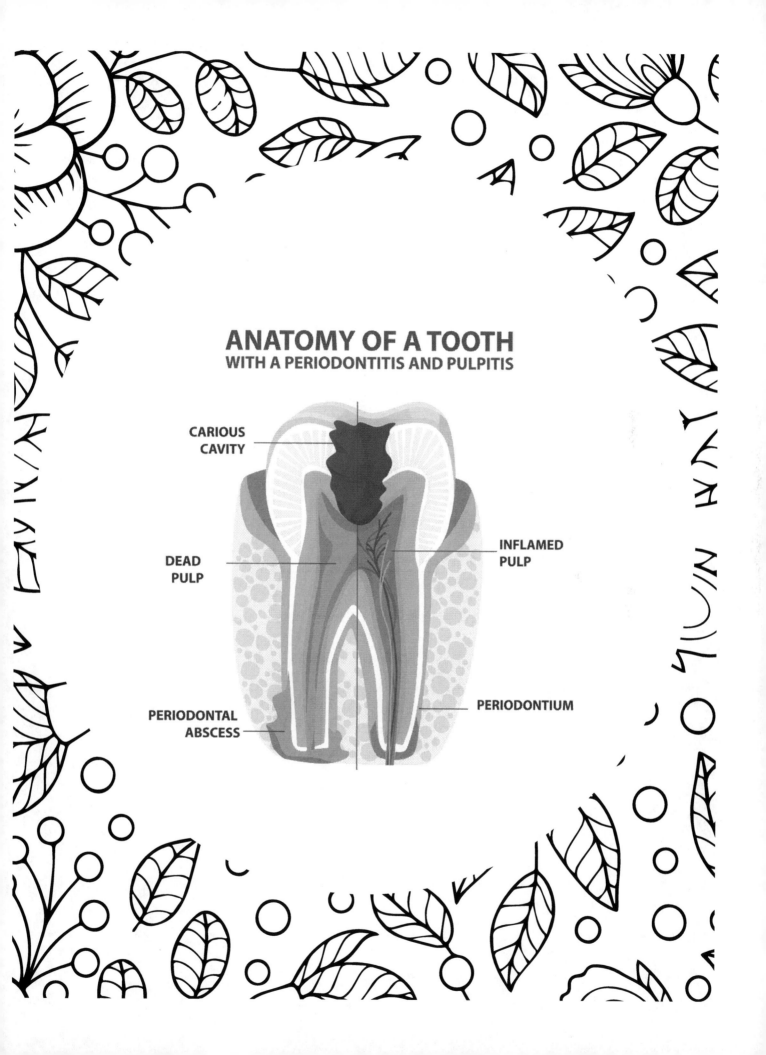

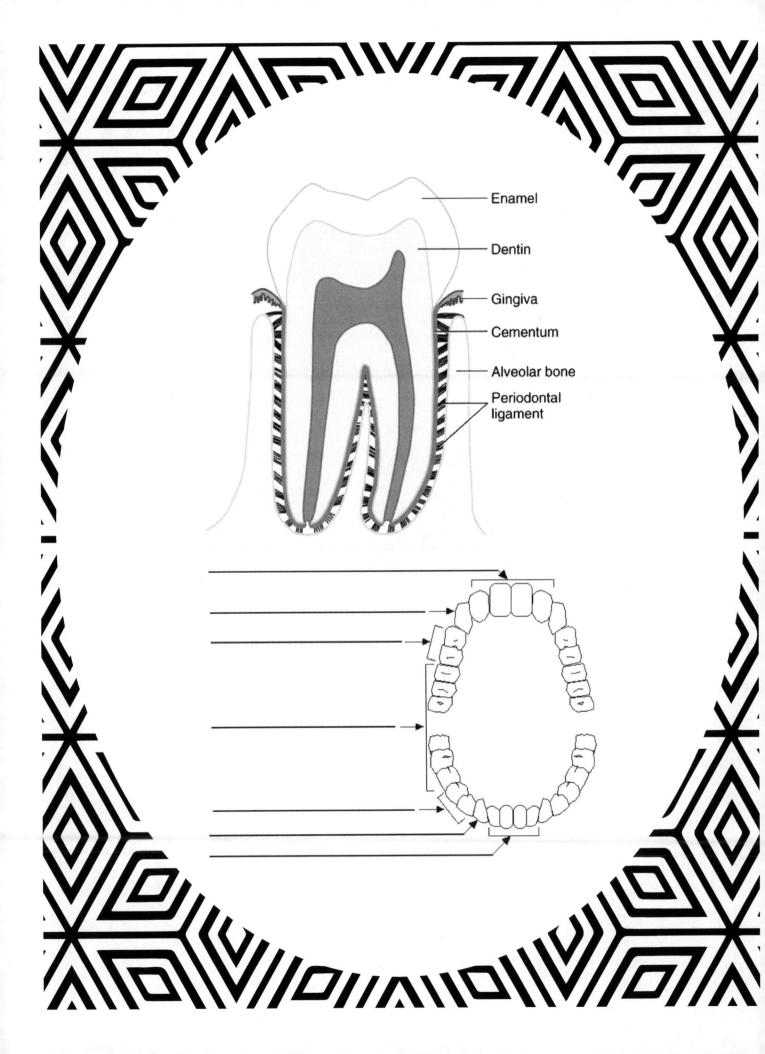

Enamel

Dentin

Gingiva

Cementum

Alveolar bone

Periodontal ligament

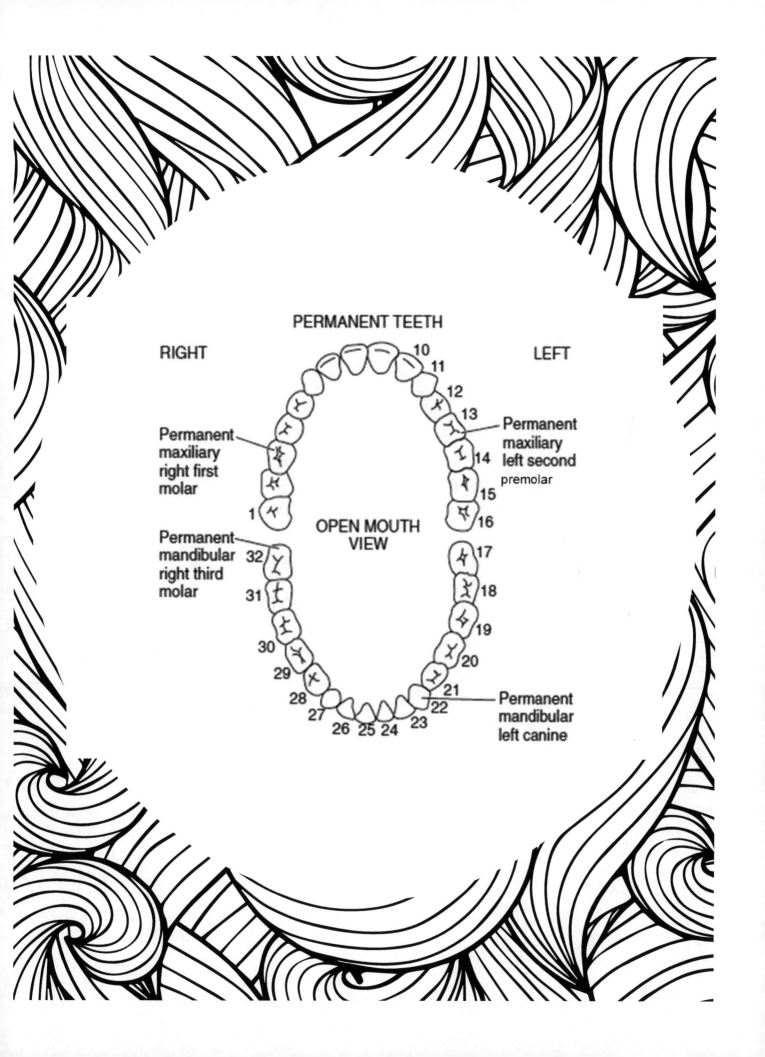

PERMANENT TEETH

RIGHT

LEFT

Permanent
maxiliary
right first
molar

Permanent
maxiliary
left second
premolar

Permanent
mandibular
right third
molar

OPEN MOUTH
VIEW

Permanent
mandibular
left canine

1
10
11
12
13
14
15
16
17
18
19
20
21
22
23
24
25
26
27
28
29
30
31
32

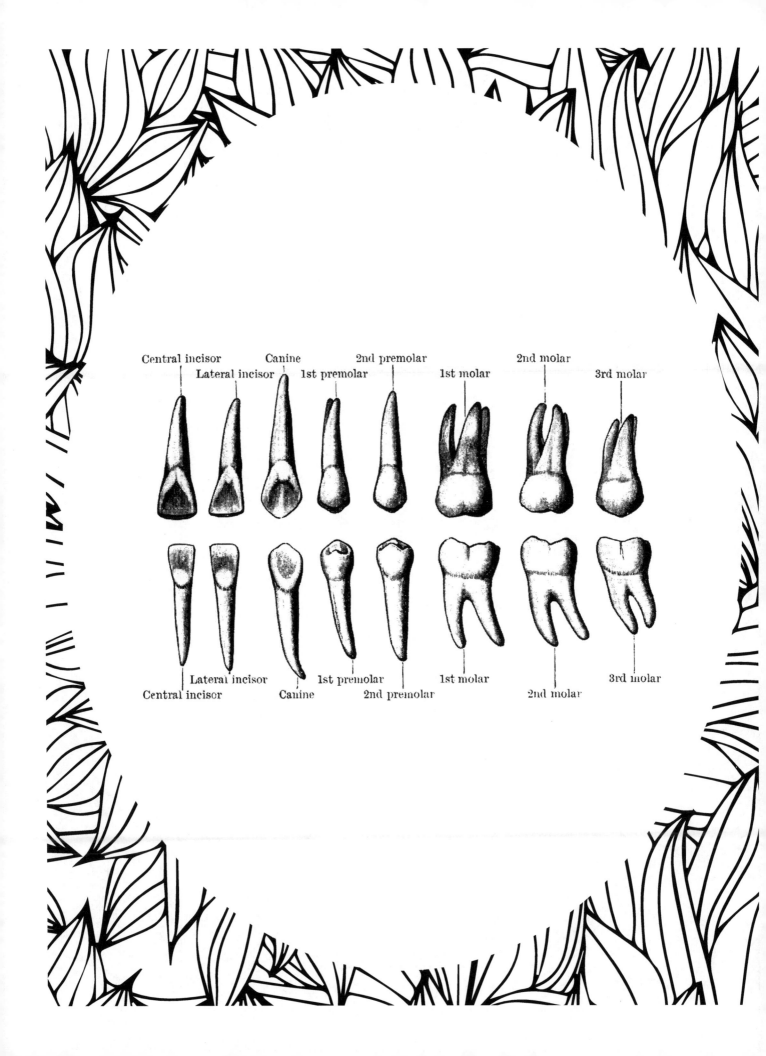

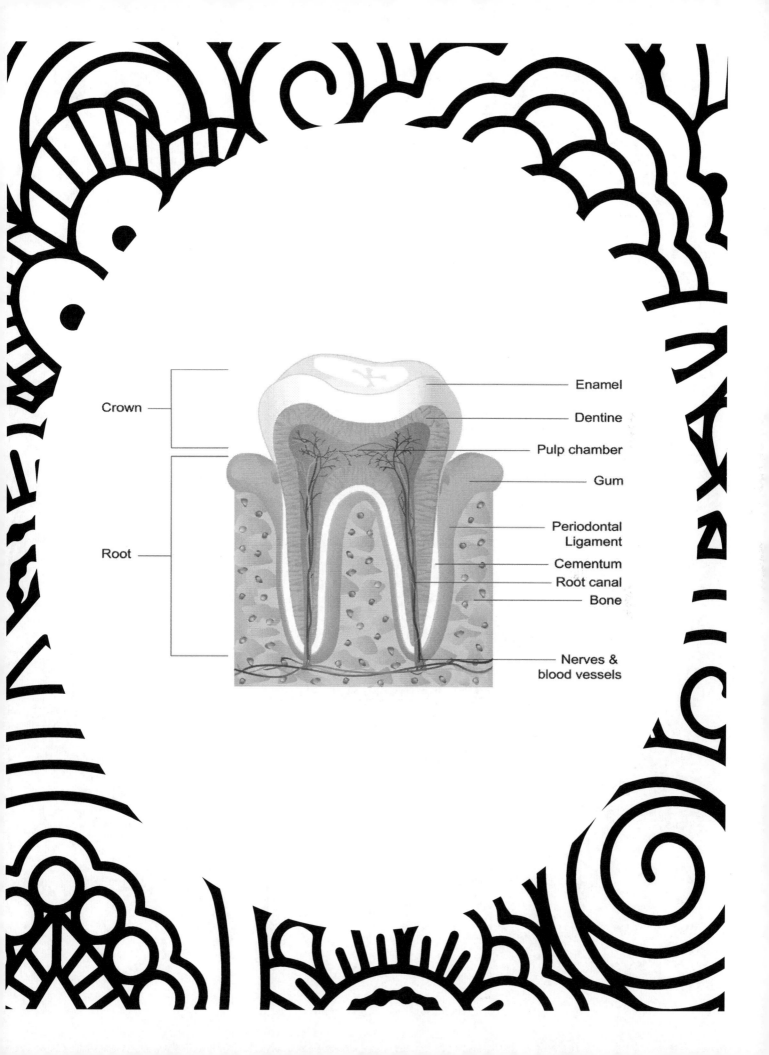

Crown

Root

Enamel

Dentine

Pulp chamber

Gum

Periodontal Ligament

Cementum

Root canal

Bone

Nerves & blood vessels

Tooth Anatomy

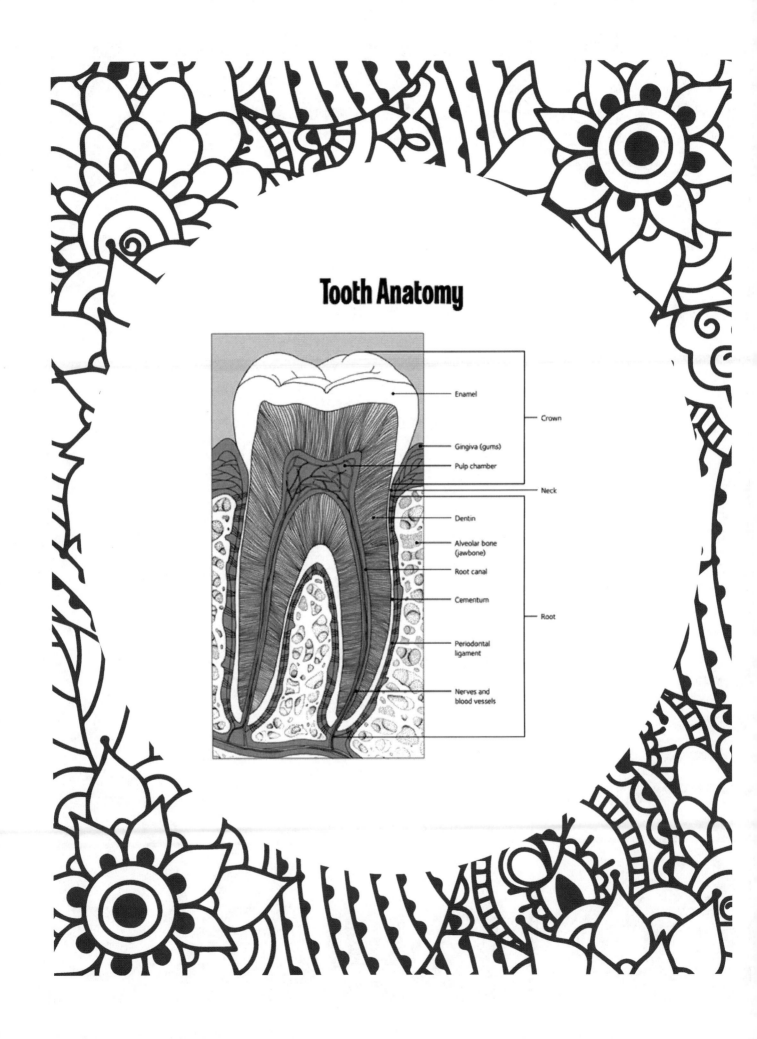

Anatomy of the tooth

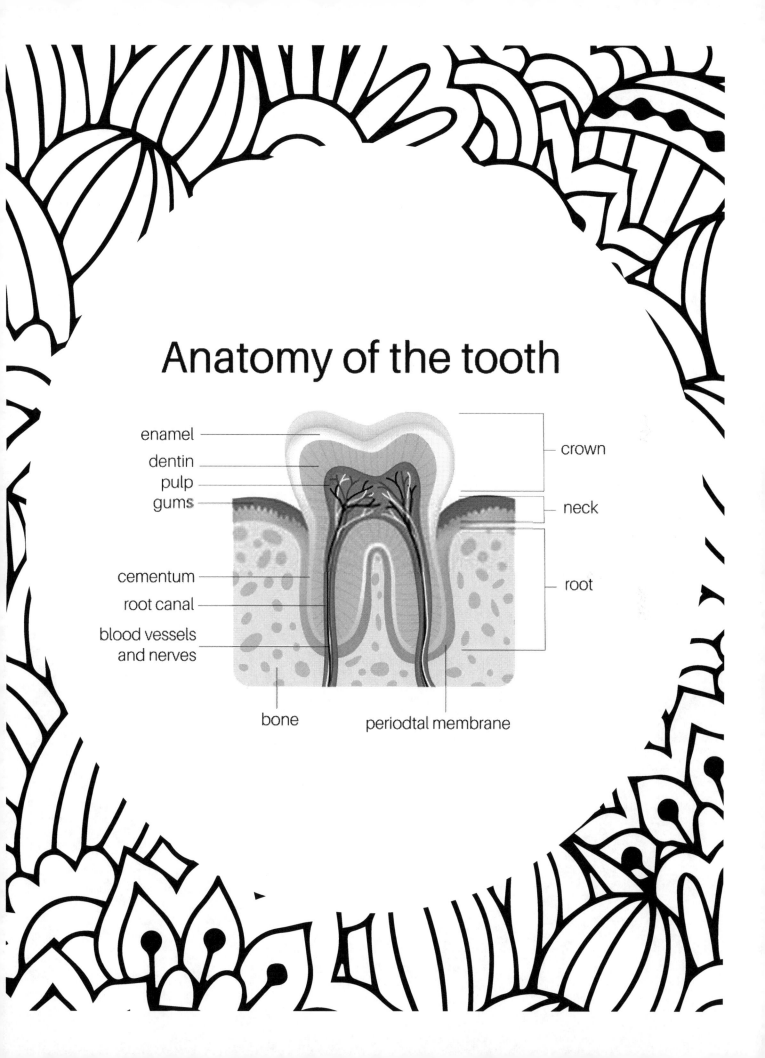

enamel

dentin

pulp

gums

crown

neck

root

cementum

root canal

blood vessels
and nerves

bone   periodtal membrane

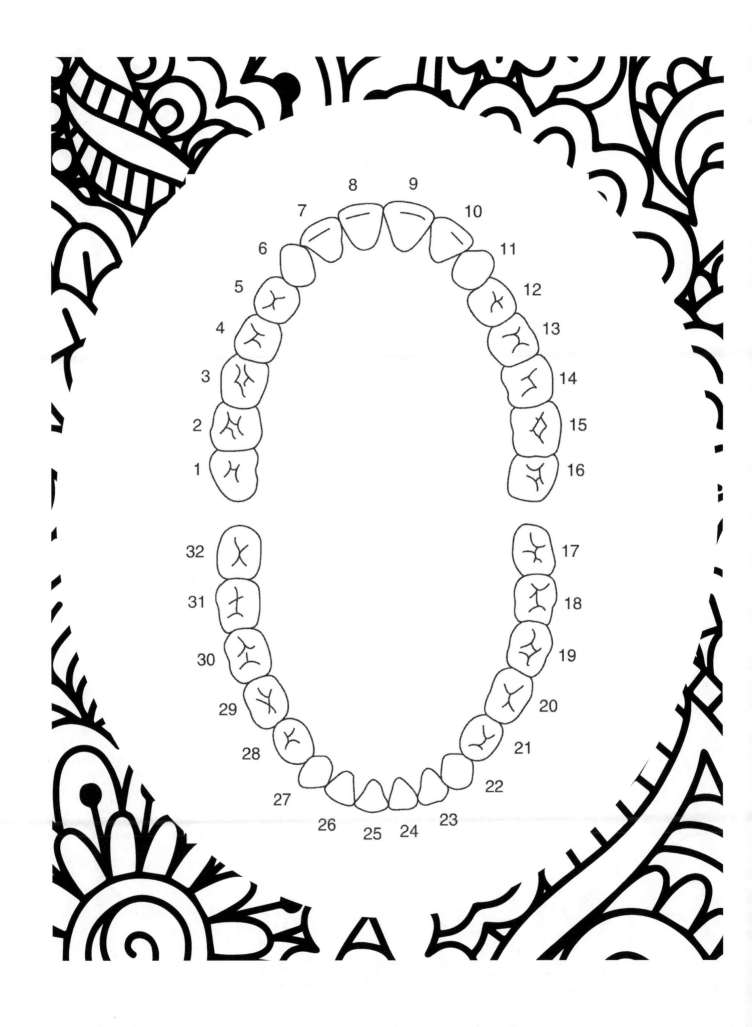

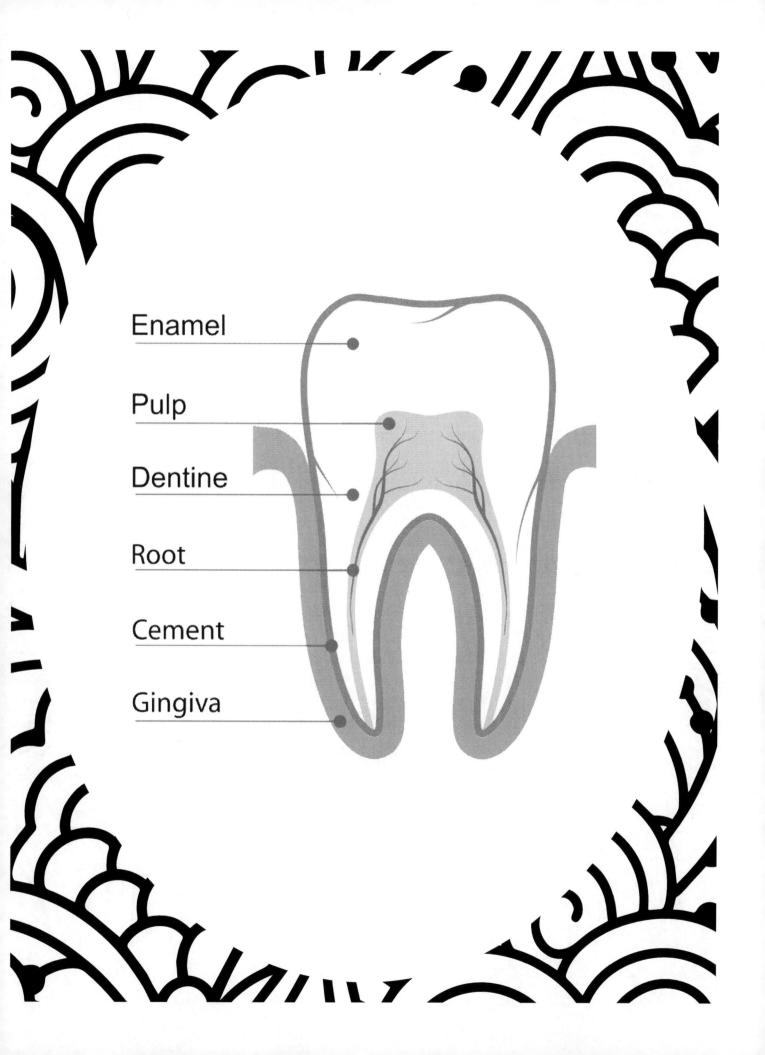

Enamel

Pulp

Dentine

Root

Cement

Gingiva

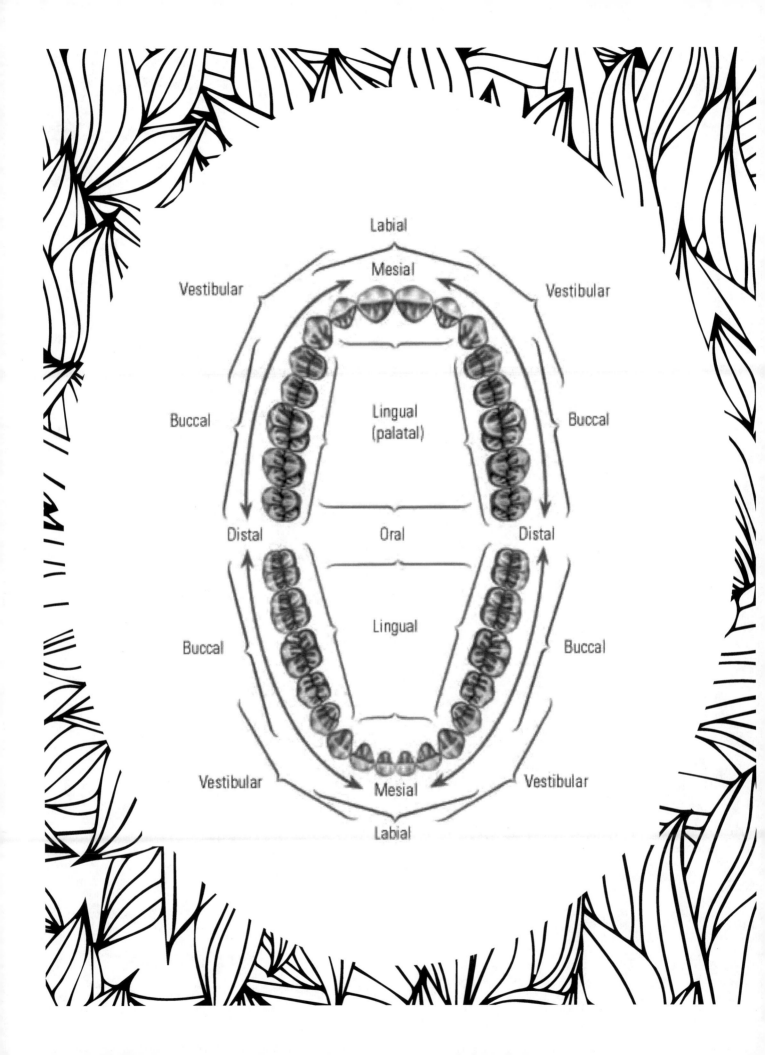

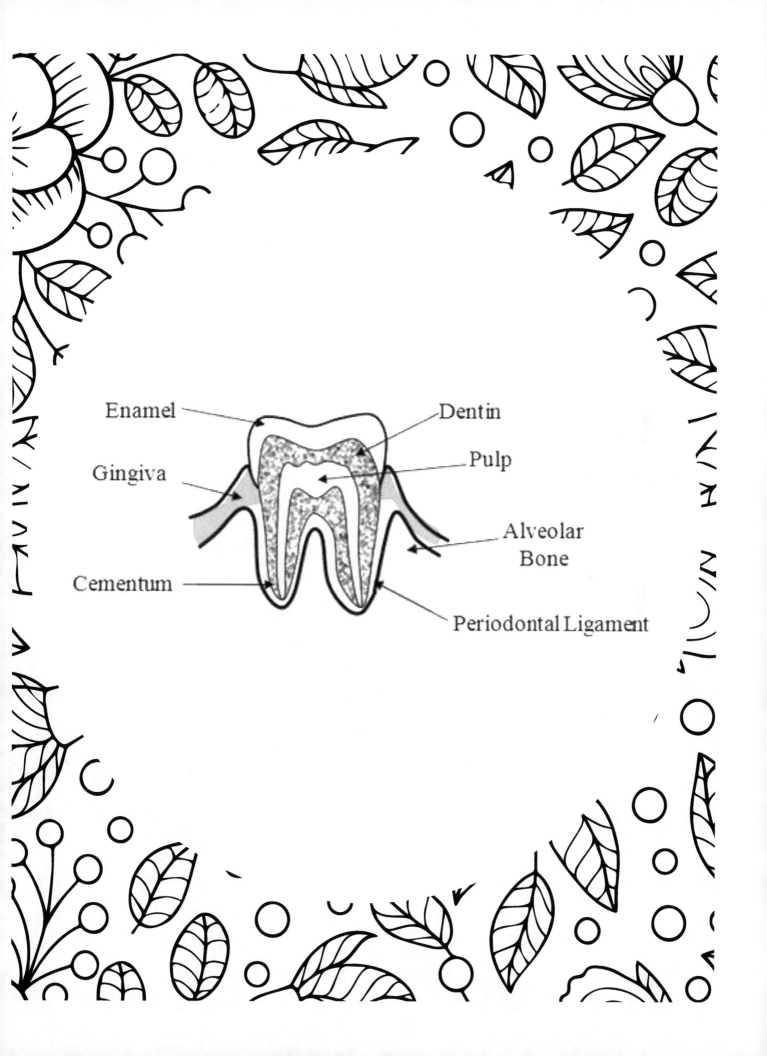

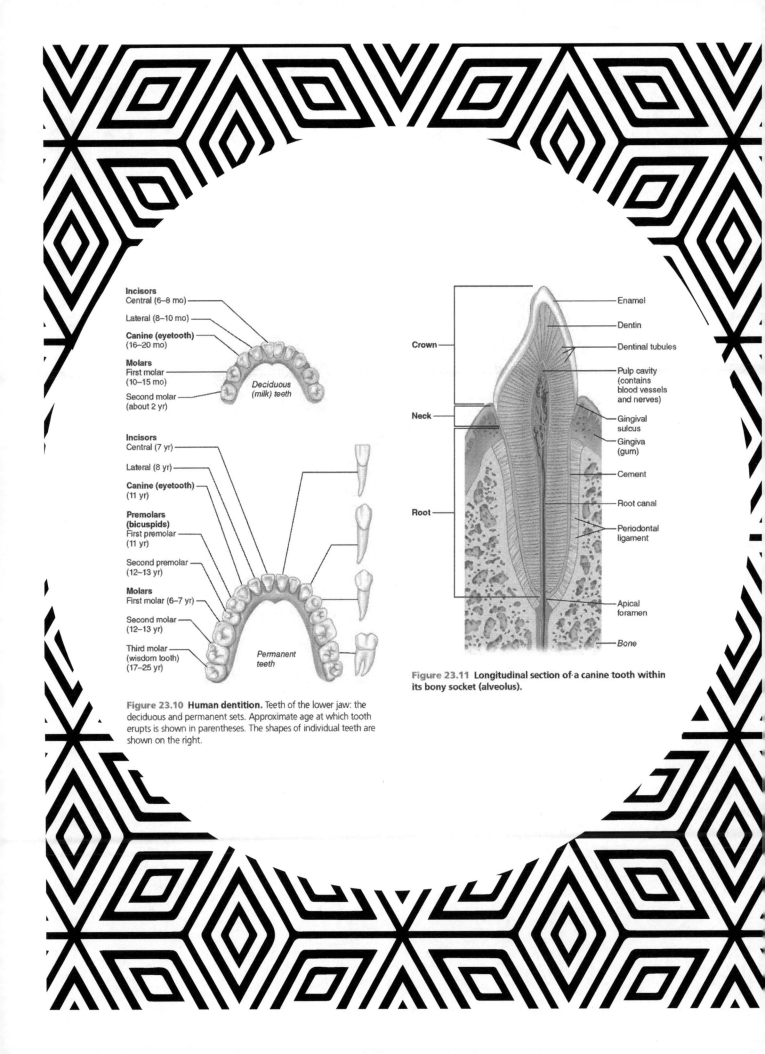

Incisors
Central (6–8 mo)
Lateral (8–10 mo)

Canine (eyetooth)
(16–20 mo)

Molars
First molar
(10–15 mo)
Second molar
(about 2 yr)

*Deciduous
(milk) teeth*

Incisors
Central (7 yr)
Lateral (8 yr)

Canine (eyetooth)
(11 yr)

**Premolars
(bicuspids)**
First premolar
(11 yr)

Second premolar
(12–13 yr)

Molars
First molar (6–7 yr)
Second molar
(12–13 yr)
Third molar
(wisdom tooth)
(17–25 yr)

*Permanent
teeth*

Figure 23.10 Human dentition. Teeth of the lower jaw: the deciduous and permanent sets. Approximate age at which tooth erupts is shown in parentheses. The shapes of individual teeth are shown on the right.

Crown
Neck
Root

Enamel
Dentin
Dentinal tubules
Pulp cavity (contains blood vessels and nerves)
Gingival sulcus
Gingiva (gum)
Cement
Root canal
Periodontal ligament
Apical foramen
Bone

Figure 23.11 Longitudinal section of a canine tooth within its bony socket (alveolus).

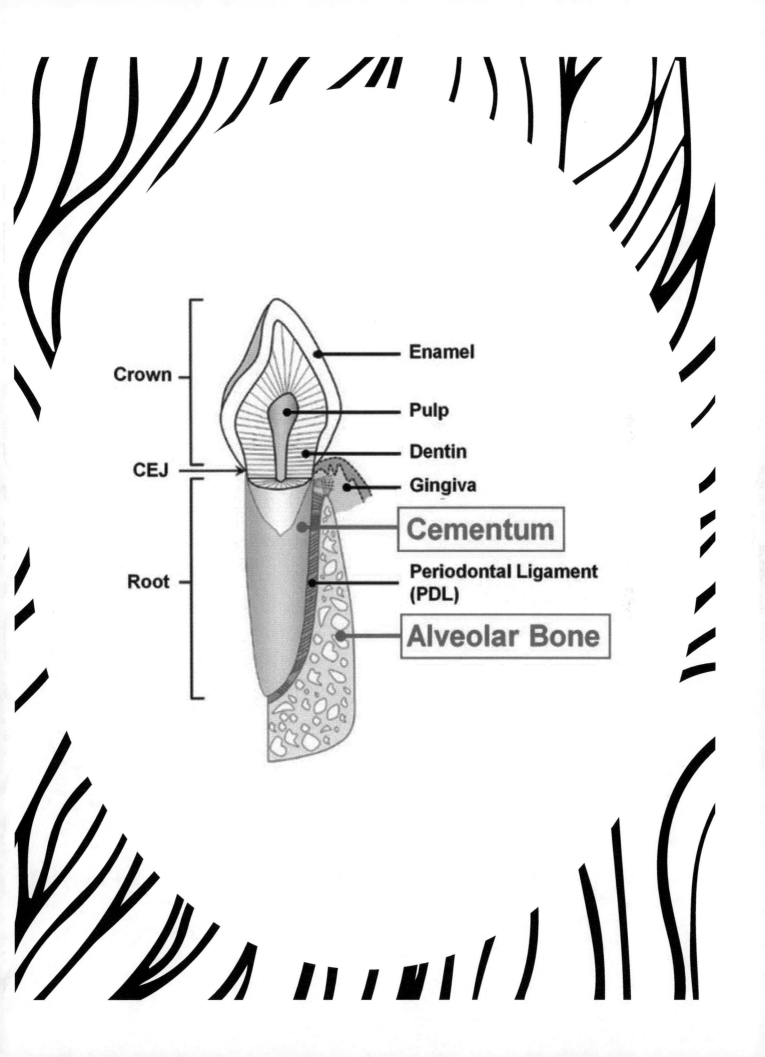

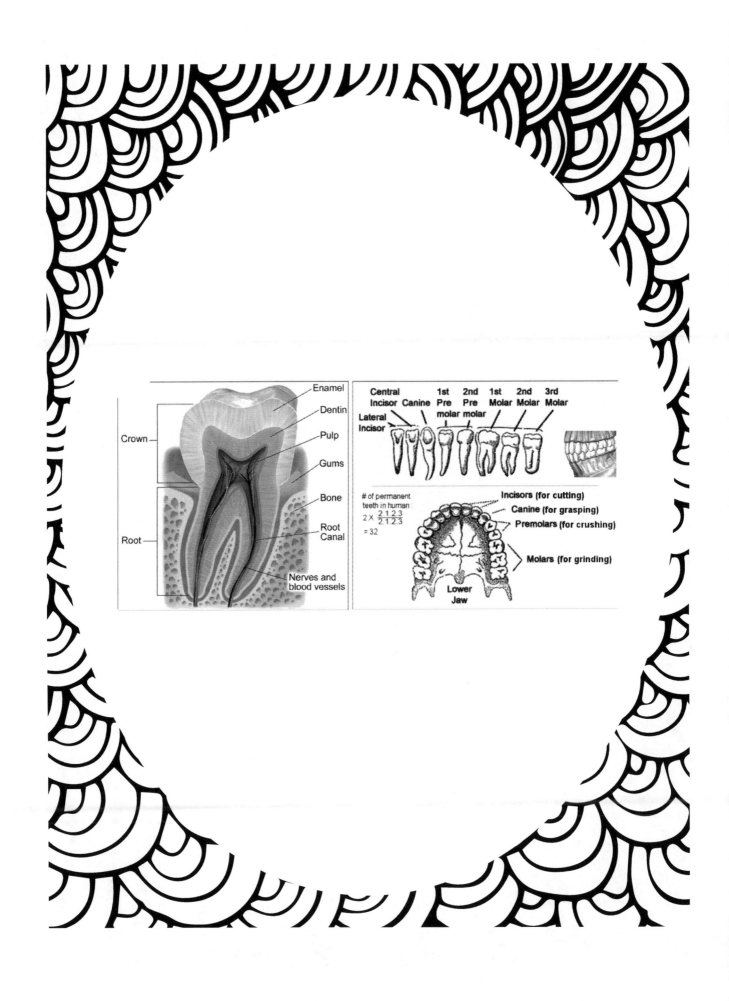

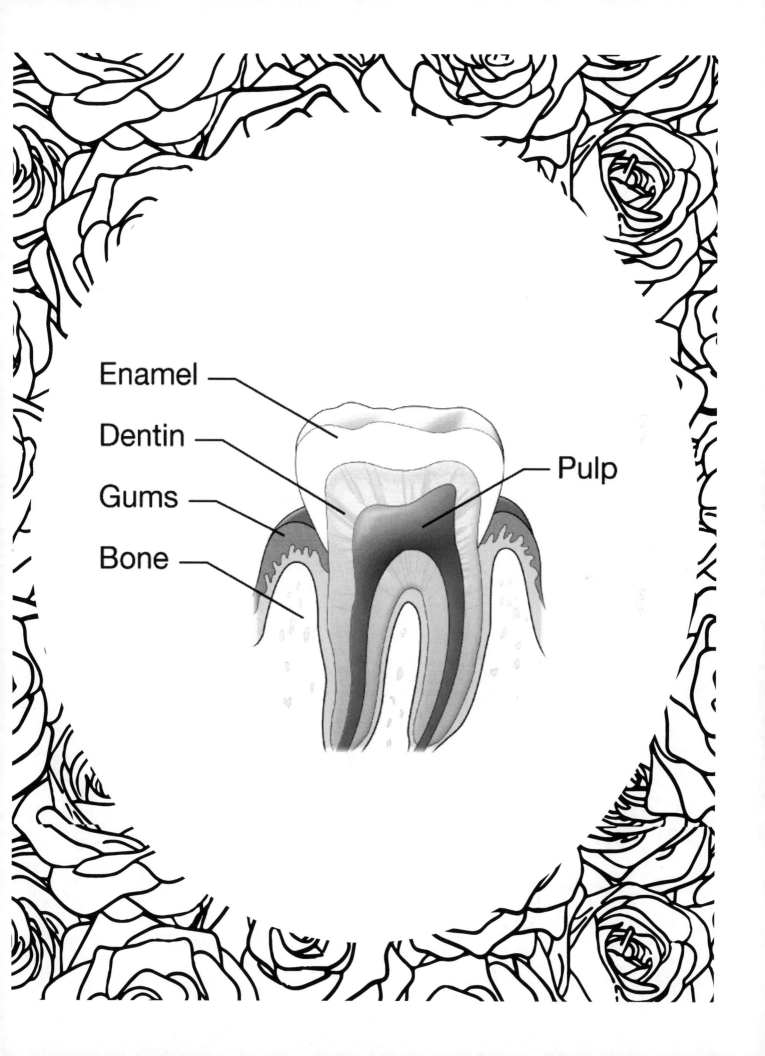

Enamel

Dentin

Gums

Bone

Pulp

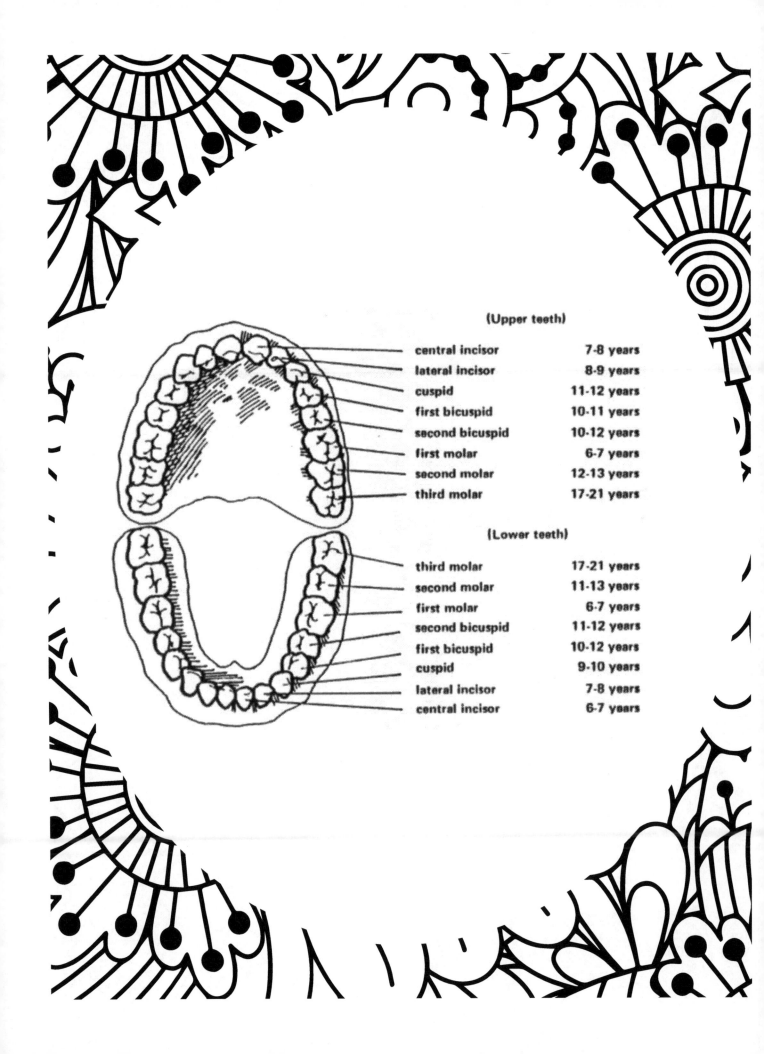

(Upper teeth)

central incisor	7-8 years
lateral incisor	8-9 years
cuspid	11-12 years
first bicuspid	10-11 years
second bicuspid	10-12 years
first molar	6-7 years
second molar	12-13 years
third molar	17-21 years

(Lower teeth)

third molar	17-21 years
second molar	11-13 years
first molar	6-7 years
second bicuspid	11-12 years
first bicuspid	10-12 years
cuspid	9-10 years
lateral incisor	7-8 years
central incisor	6-7 years

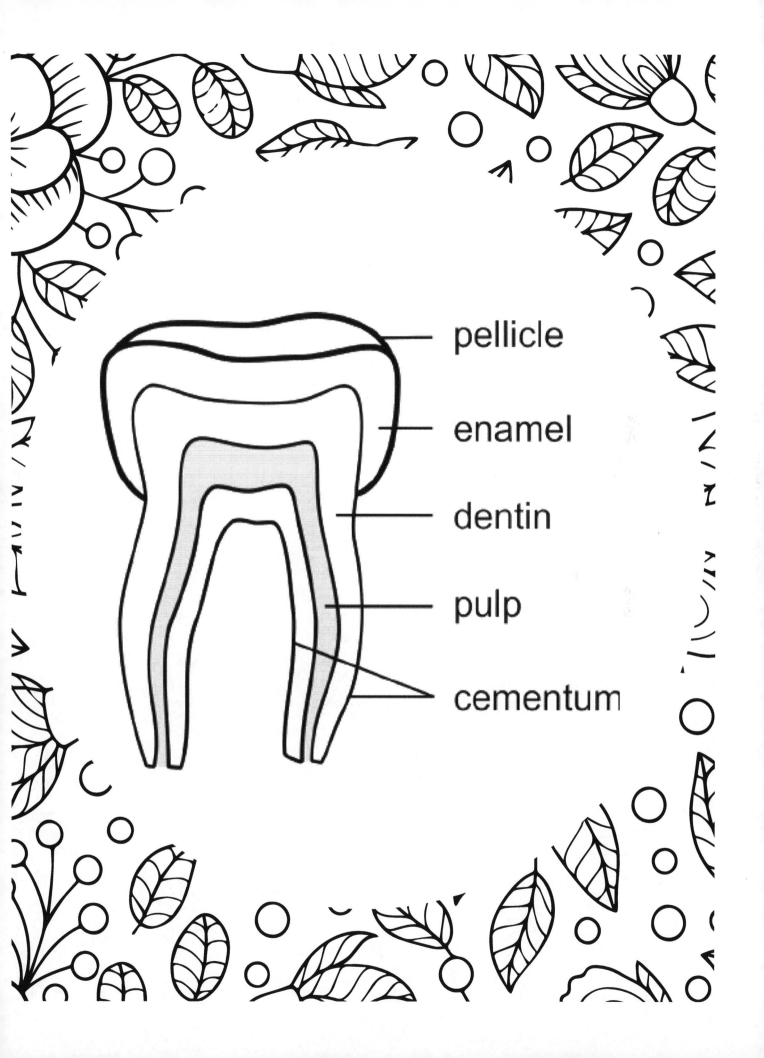

pellicle

enamel

dentin

pulp

cementum

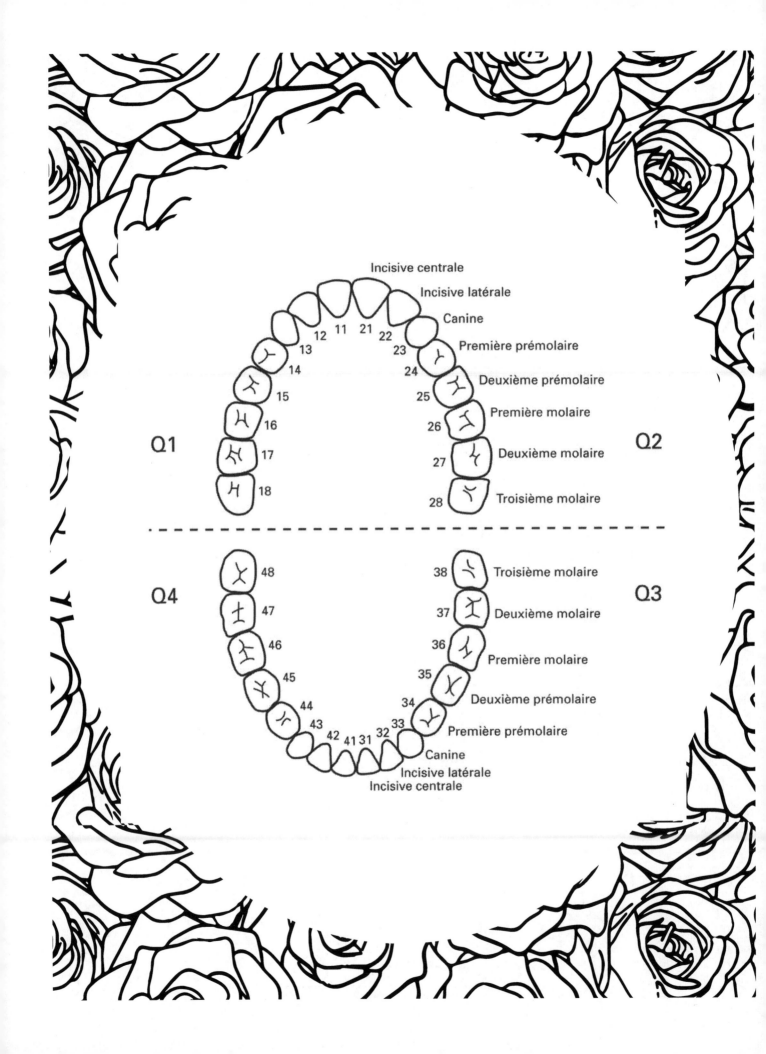

Incisive centrale
Incisive latérale
Canine
Première prémolaire
Deuxième prémolaire
Première molaire
Deuxième molaire
Troisième molaire

Q1
Q2
Q4
Q3

12 11 21 22
13 23
14 24
15 25
16 26
17 27
18 28

48 38 Troisième molaire
47 37 Deuxième molaire
46 36 Première molaire
45 35
44 34 Deuxième prémolaire
43 33 Première prémolaire
42 41 31 32
Canine
Incisive latérale
Incisive centrale

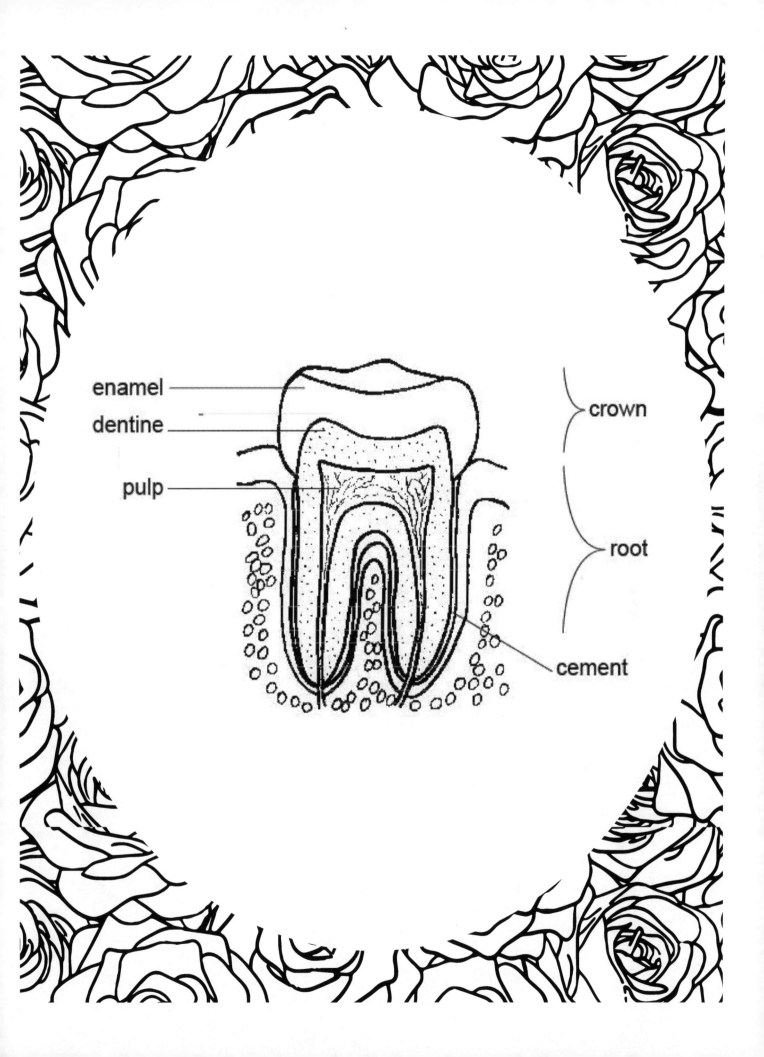

enamel

dentine

pulp

crown

root

cement

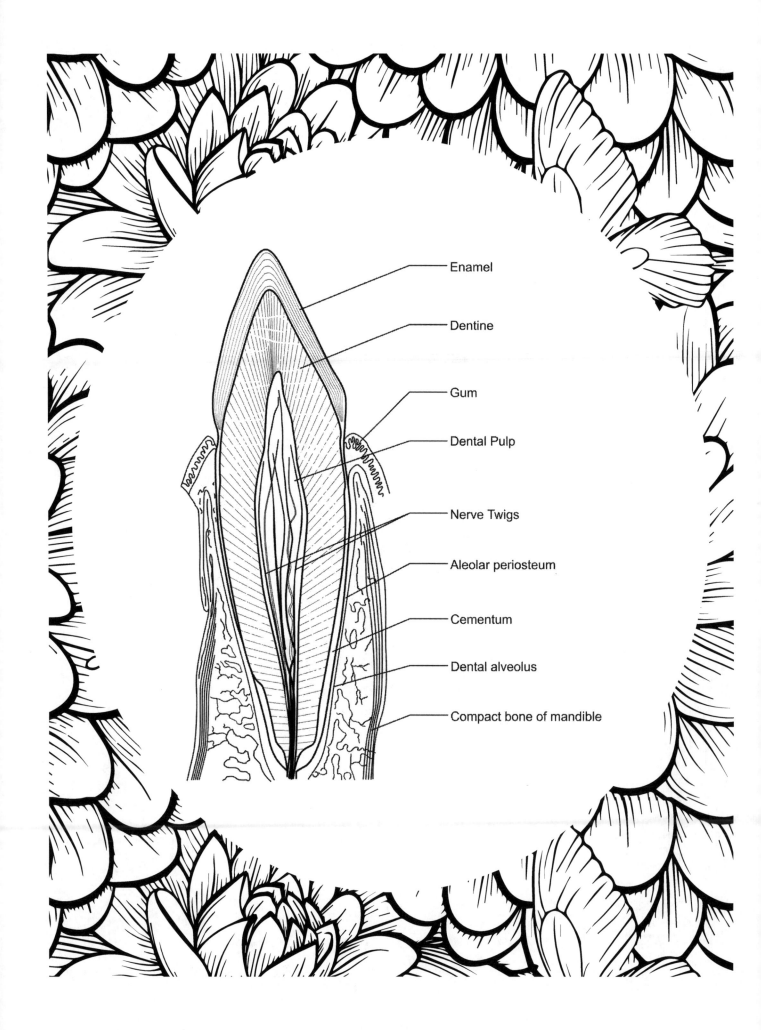

Enamel

Dentine

Gum

Dental Pulp

Nerve Twigs

Aleolar periosteum

Cementum

Dental alveolus

Compact bone of mandible

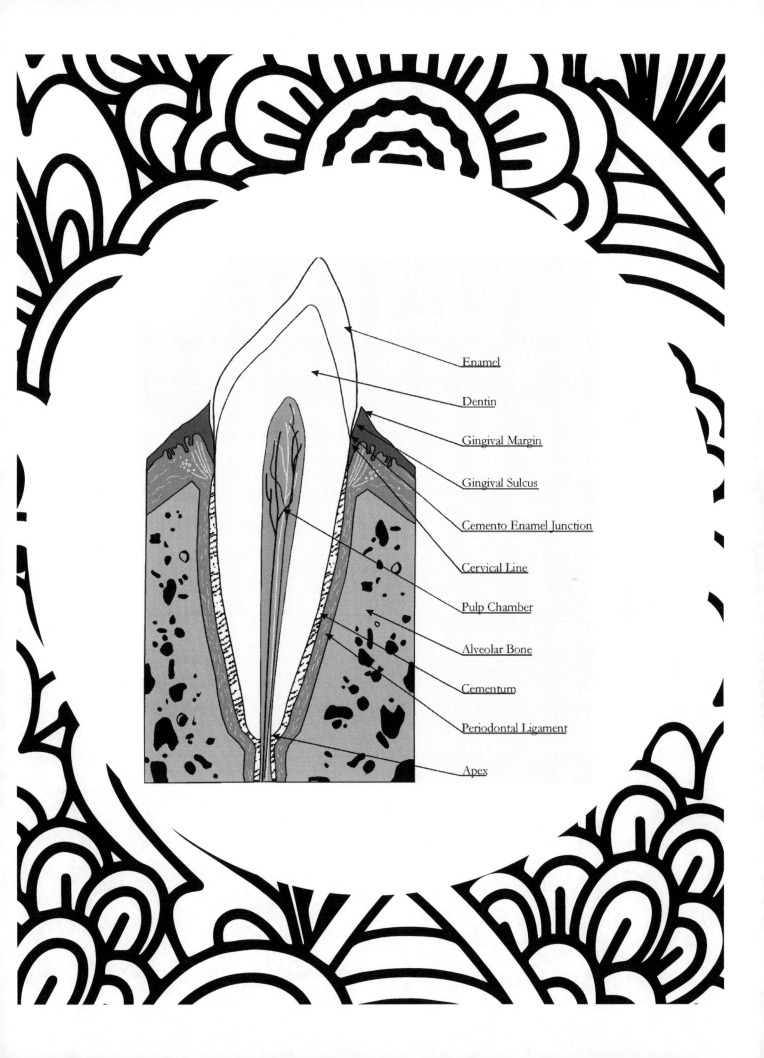

Enamel

Dentin

Gingival Margin

Gingival Sulcus

Cemento Enamel Junction

Cervical Line

Pulp Chamber

Alveolar Bone

Cementum

Periodontal Ligament

Apex

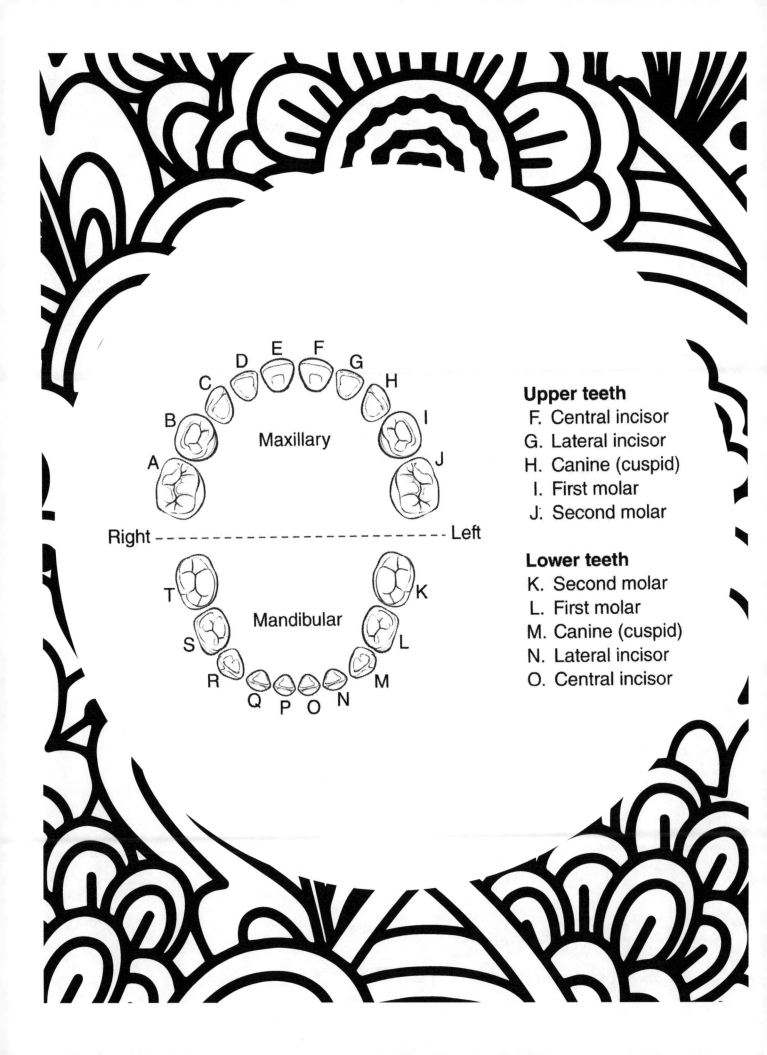

Maxillary

Right - Left

Mandibular

Upper teeth
F. Central incisor
G. Lateral incisor
H. Canine (cuspid)
I. First molar
J. Second molar

Lower teeth
K. Second molar
L. First molar
M. Canine (cuspid)
N. Lateral incisor
O. Central incisor

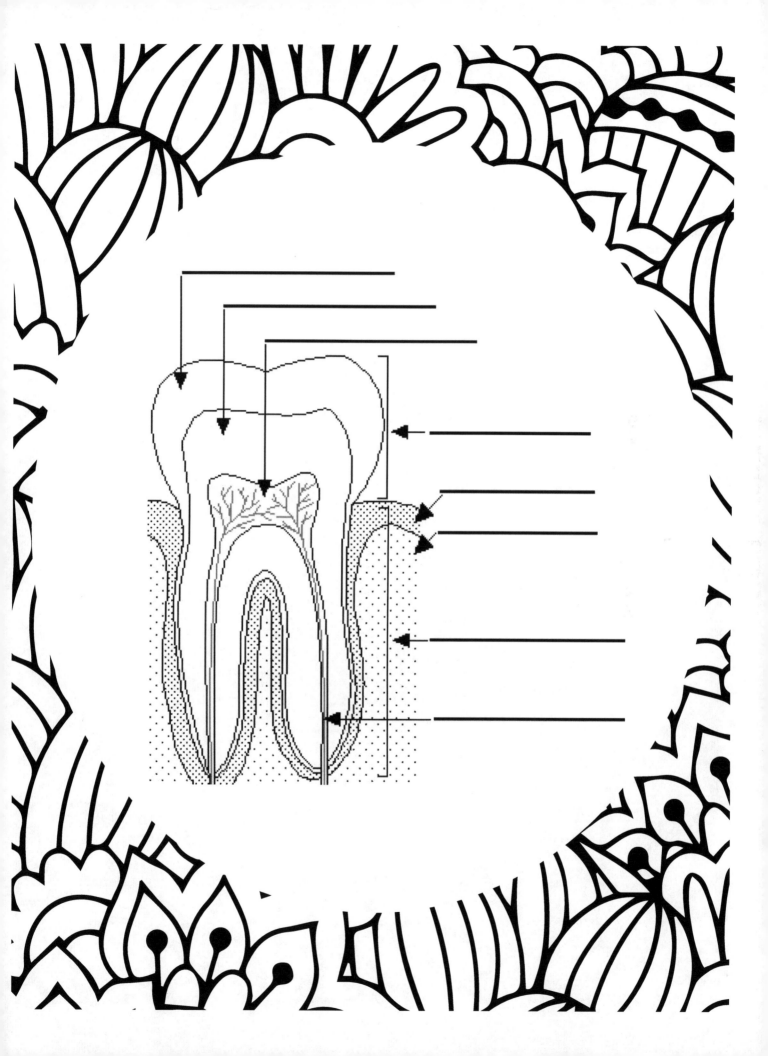

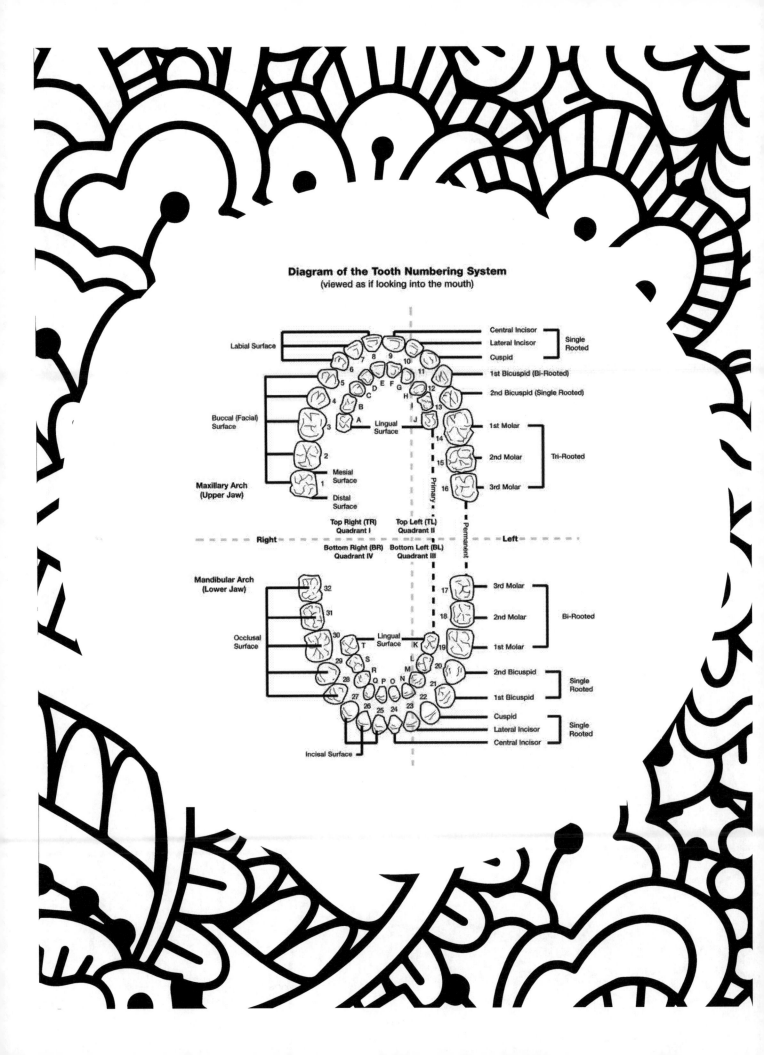

Diagram of the Tooth Numbering System
(viewed as if looking into the mouth)

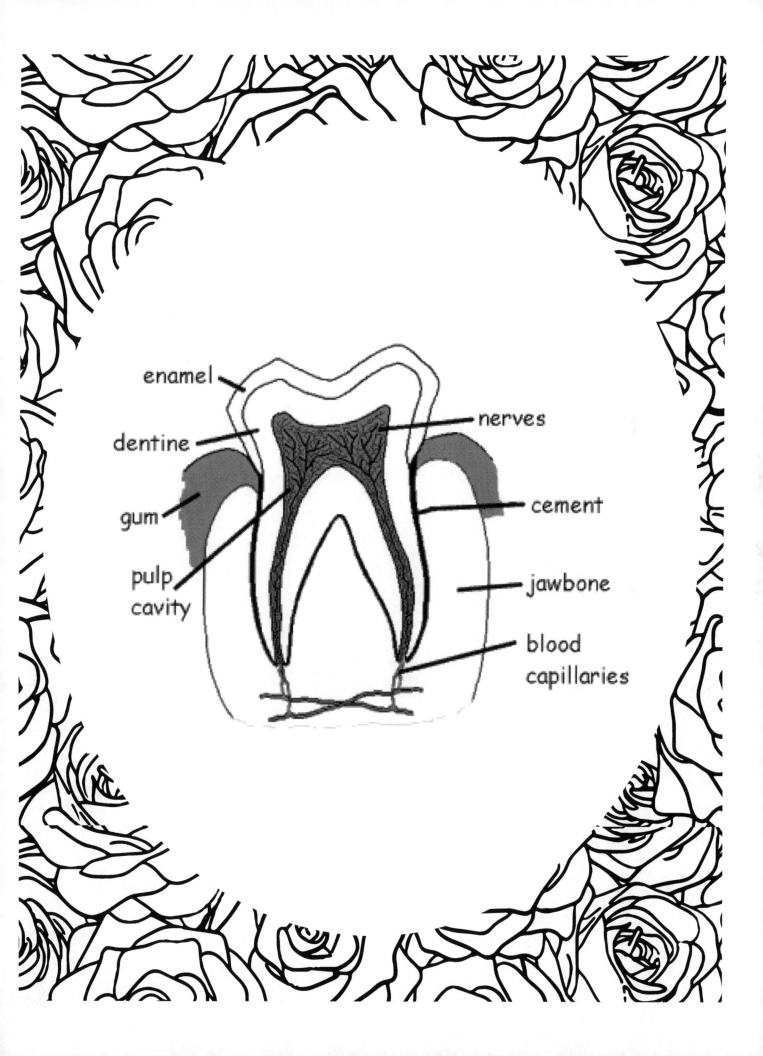

enamel

nerves

dentine

gum

cement

pulp
cavity

jawbone

blood
capillaries

The relations of the main dental tissues

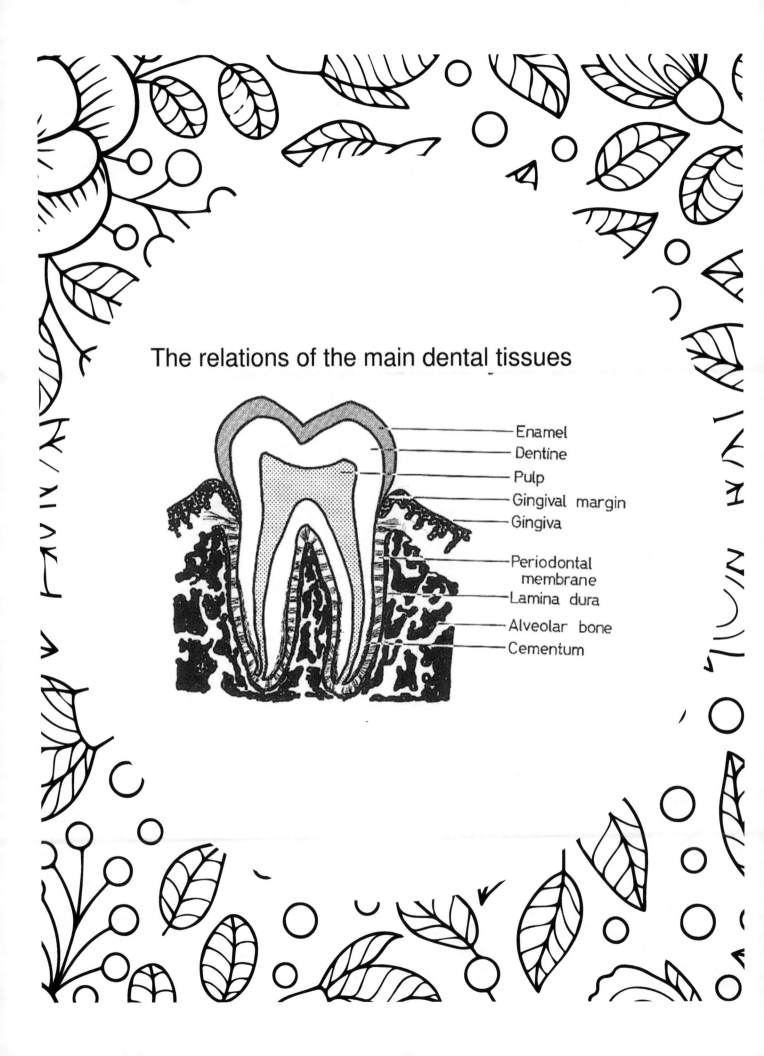

- Enamel
- Dentine
- Pulp
- Gingival margin
- Gingiva
- Periodontal membrane
- Lamina dura
- Alveolar bone
- Cementum

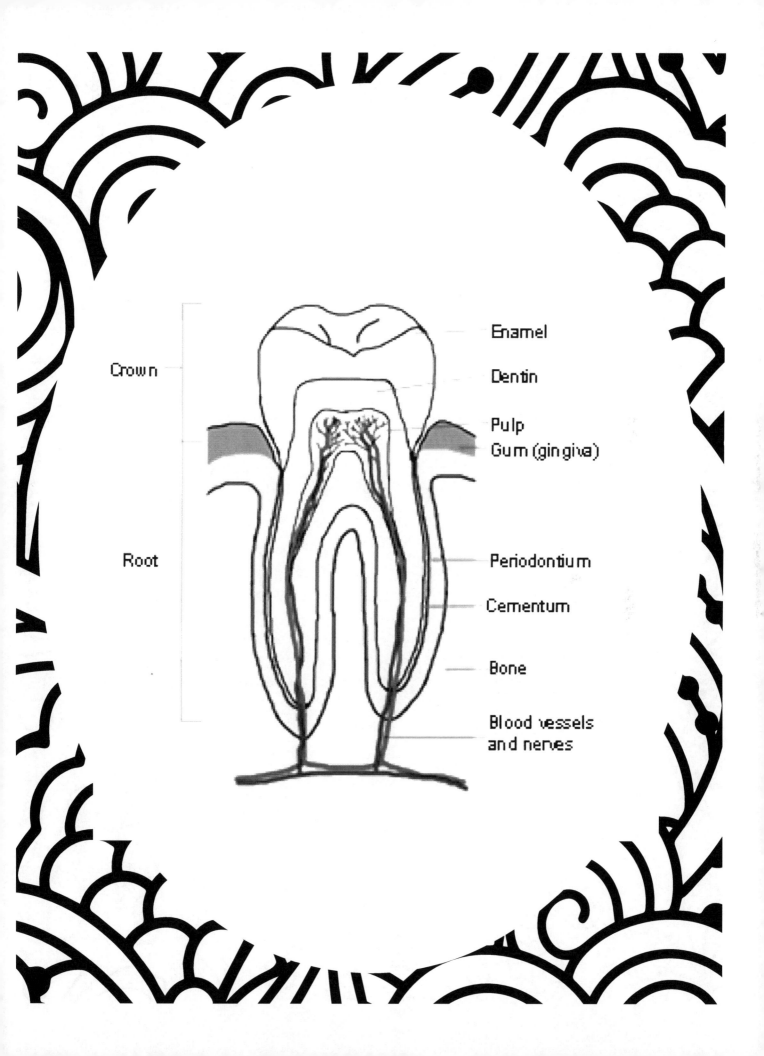

Crown

Root

Enamel

Dentin

Pulp

Gum (gingiva)

Periodontium

Cementum

Bone

Blood vessels
and nerves

Primary Teeth

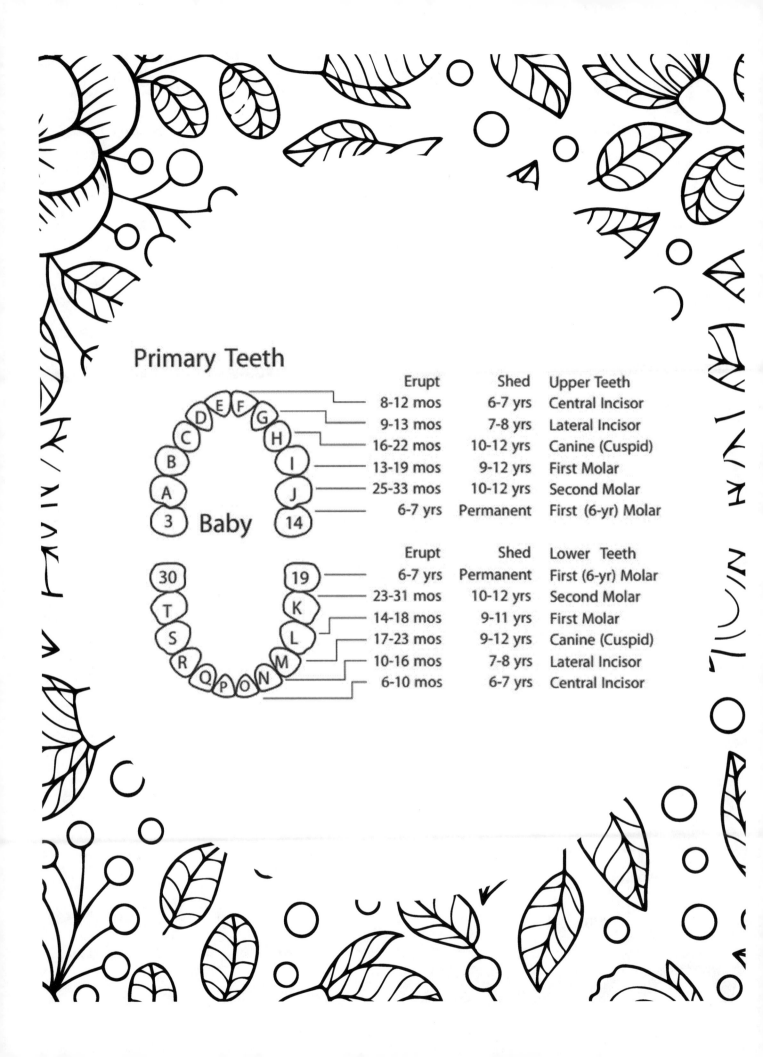

Baby

Erupt	Shed	Upper Teeth
8-12 mos	6-7 yrs	Central Incisor
9-13 mos	7-8 yrs	Lateral Incisor
16-22 mos	10-12 yrs	Canine (Cuspid)
13-19 mos	9-12 yrs	First Molar
25-33 mos	10-12 yrs	Second Molar
6-7 yrs	Permanent	First (6-yr) Molar

Erupt	Shed	Lower Teeth
6-7 yrs	Permanent	First (6-yr) Molar
23-31 mos	10-12 yrs	Second Molar
14-18 mos	9-11 yrs	First Molar
17-23 mos	9-12 yrs	Canine (Cuspid)
10-16 mos	7-8 yrs	Lateral Incisor
6-10 mos	6-7 yrs	Central Incisor

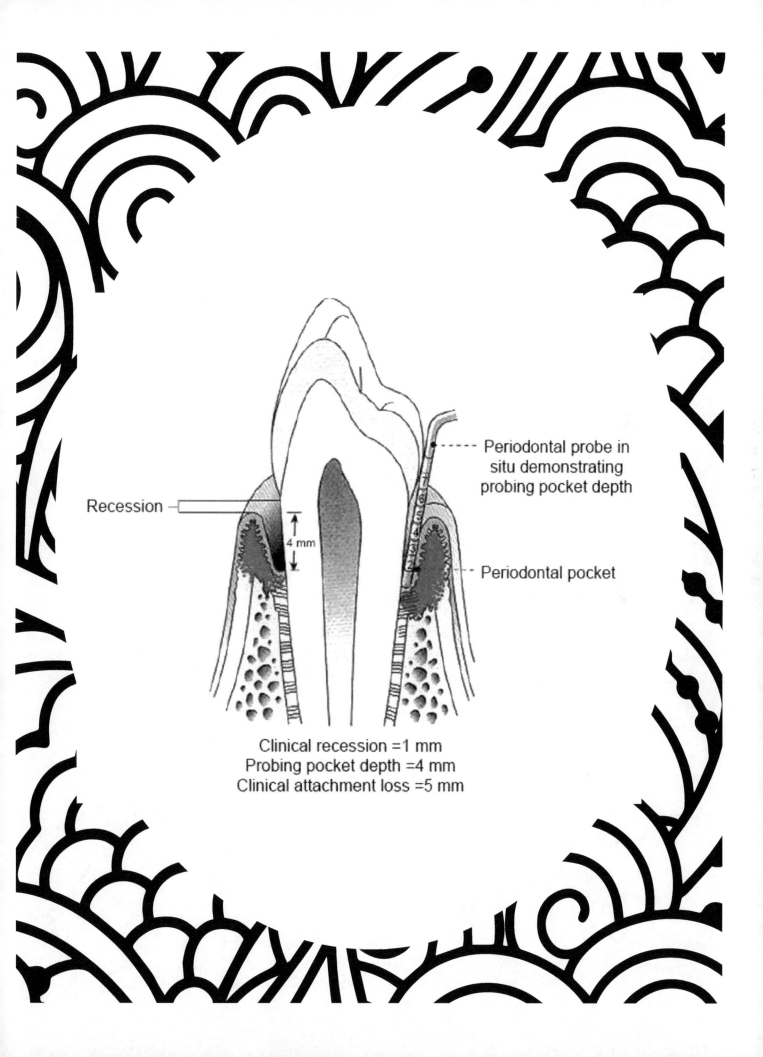

Recession

Periodontal probe in situ demonstrating probing pocket depth

4 mm

Periodontal pocket

Clinical recession =1 mm
Probing pocket depth =4 mm
Clinical attachment loss =5 mm

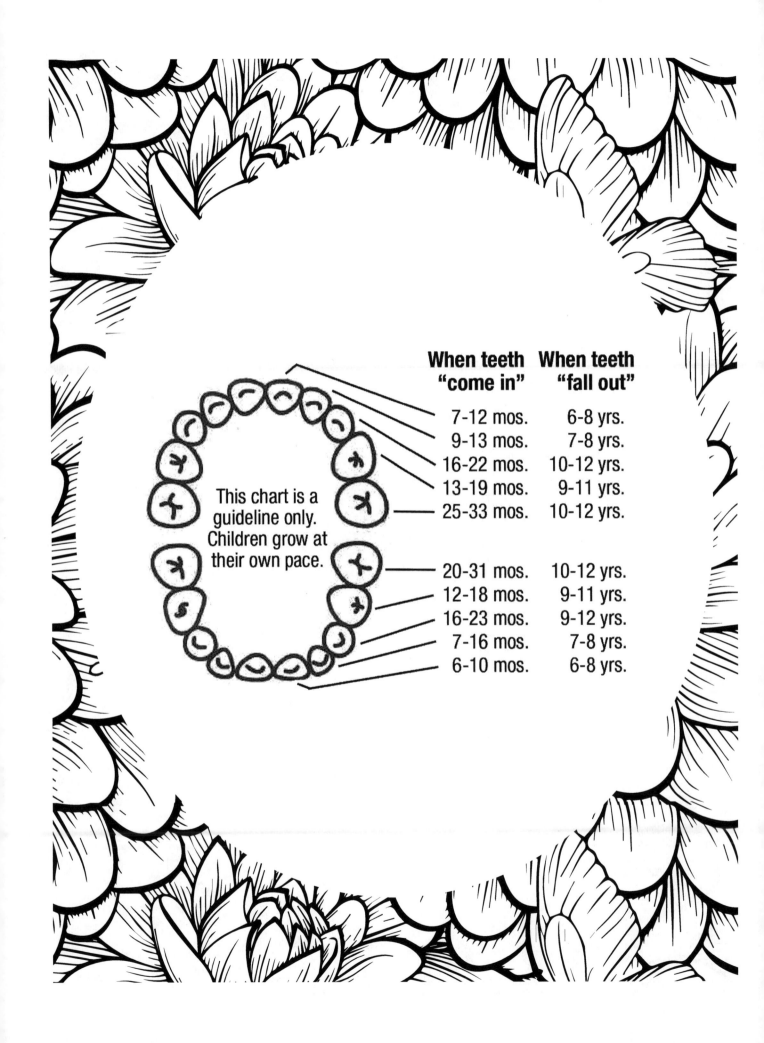

This chart is a guideline only. Children grow at their own pace.

When teeth "come in"	When teeth "fall out"
7-12 mos.	6-8 yrs.
9-13 mos.	7-8 yrs.
16-22 mos.	10-12 yrs.
13-19 mos.	9-11 yrs.
25-33 mos.	10-12 yrs.
20-31 mos.	10-12 yrs.
12-18 mos.	9-11 yrs.
16-23 mos.	9-12 yrs.
7-16 mos.	7-8 yrs.
6-10 mos.	6-8 yrs.

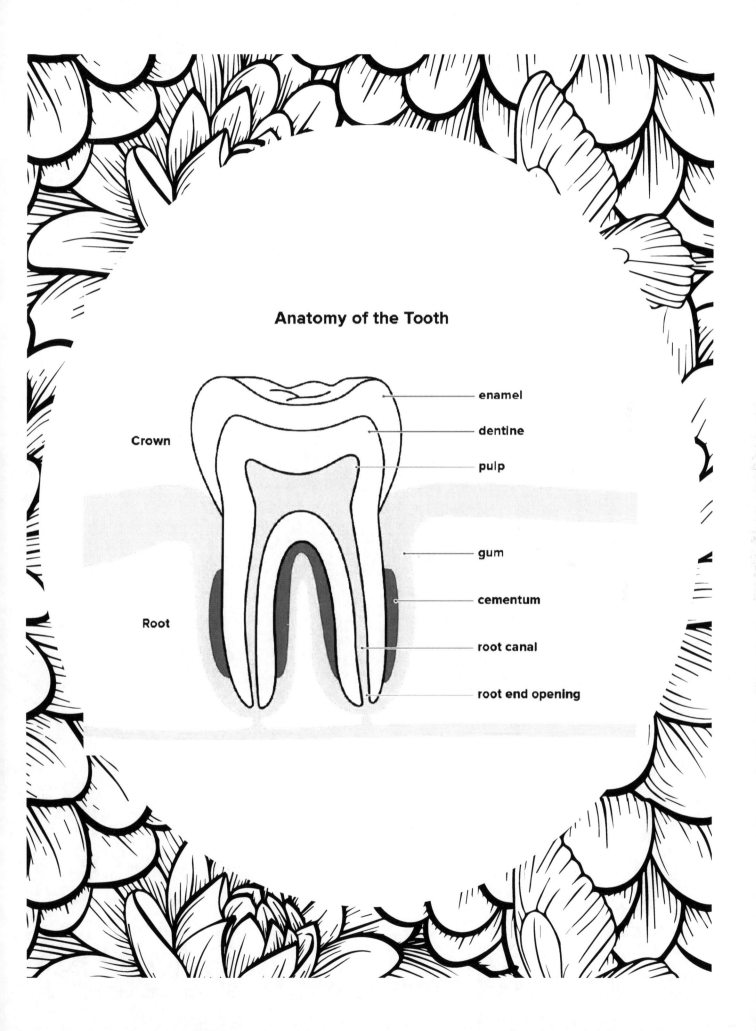

Anatomy of the Tooth

Crown

Root

enamel

dentine

pulp

gum

cementum

root canal

root end opening

TOOTH ANATOMY

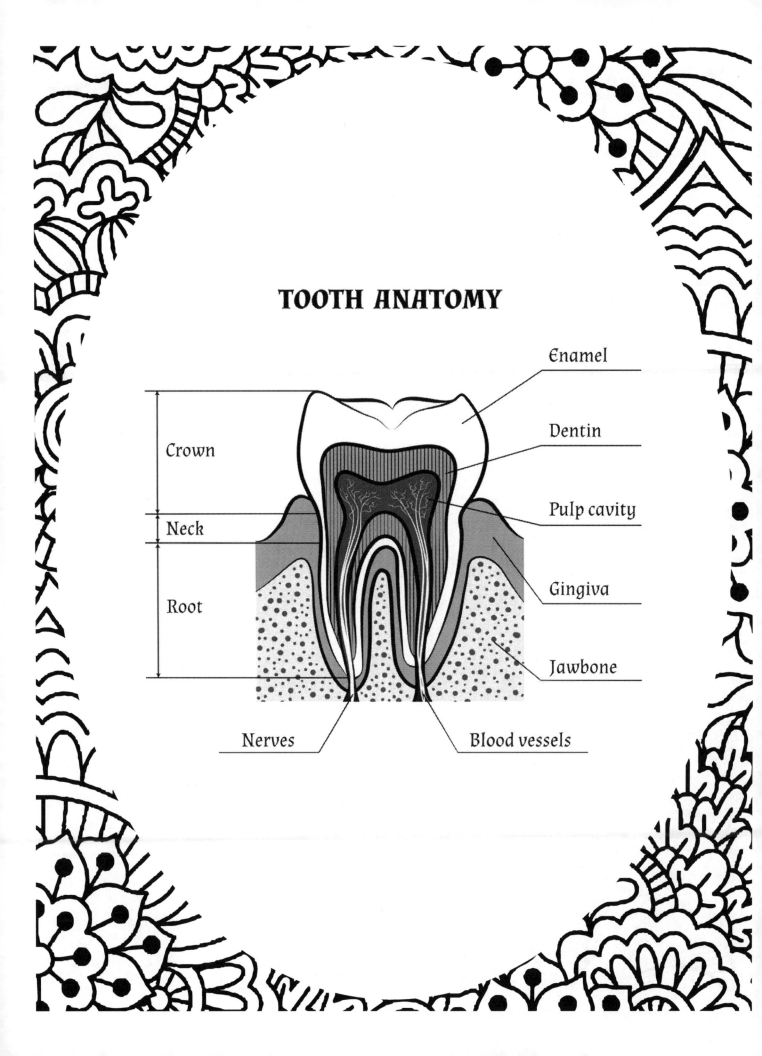

Enamel

Dentin

Pulp cavity

Gingiva

Jawbone

Crown

Neck

Root

Nerves

Blood vessels

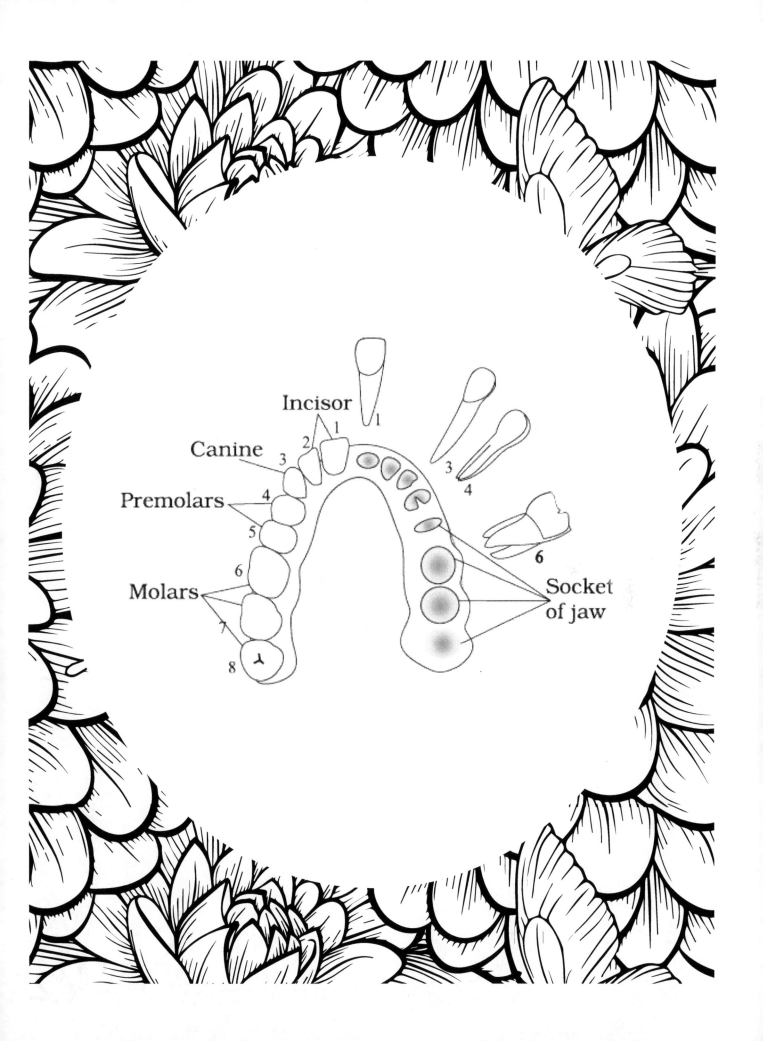

Incisor

Canine

Premolars

Molars

Socket
of jaw

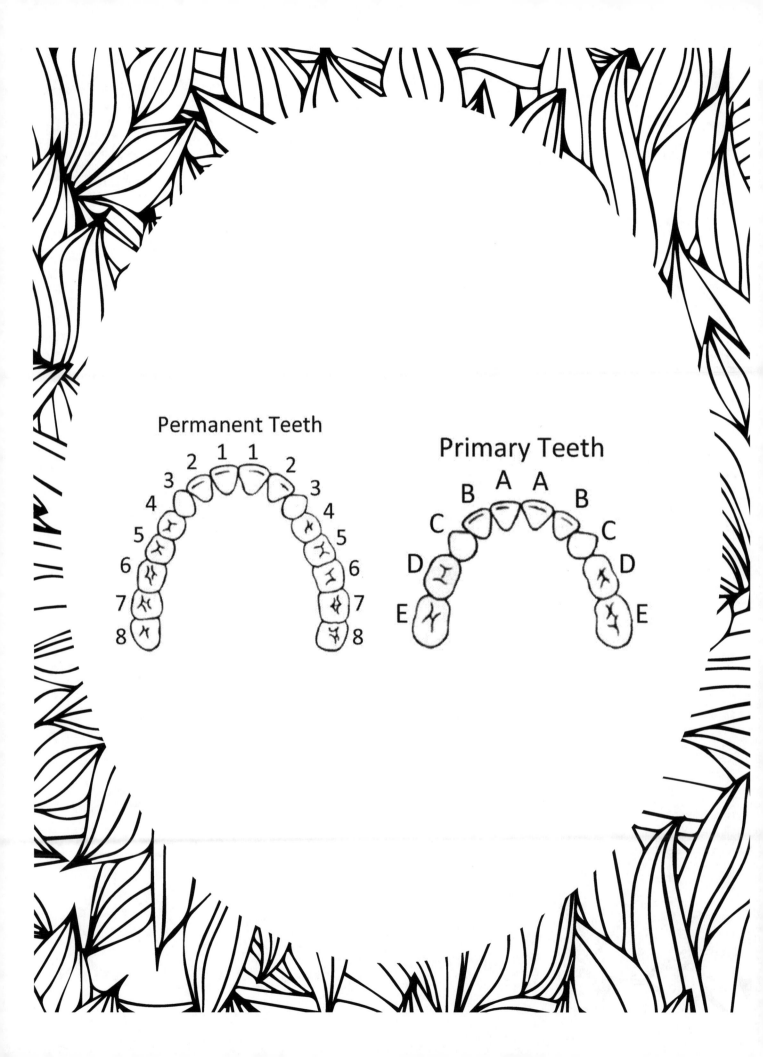

Permanent Teeth

Primary Teeth

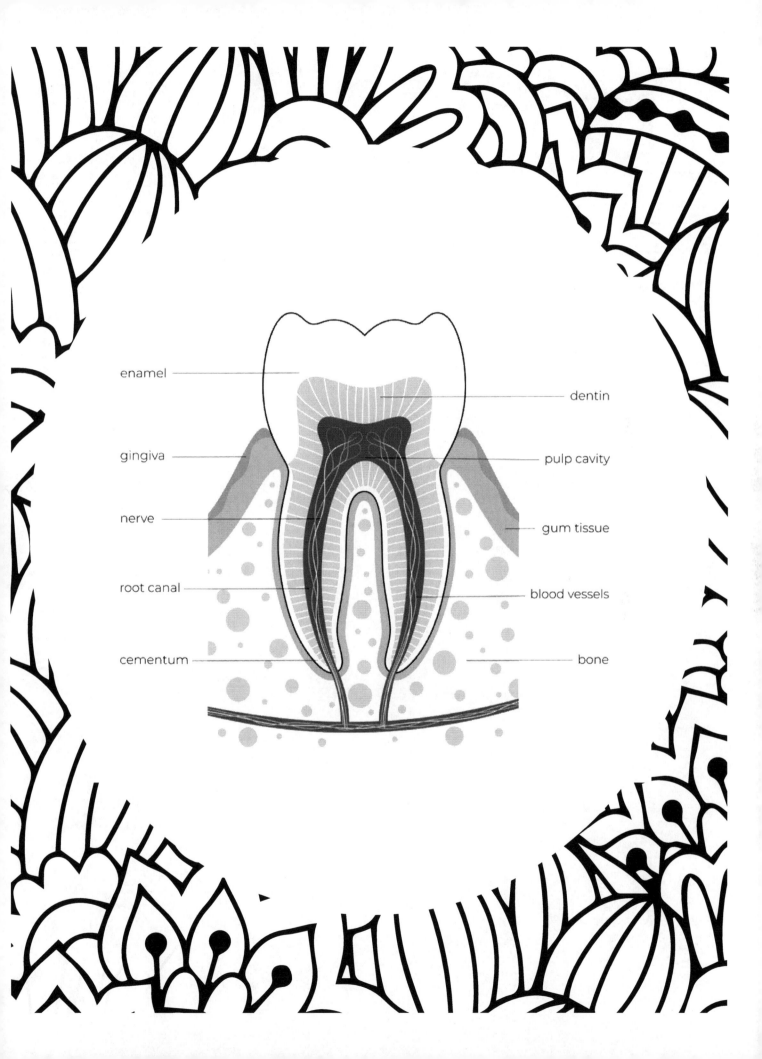

enamel

dentin

gingiva

pulp cavity

nerve

gum tissue

root canal

blood vessels

cementum

bone

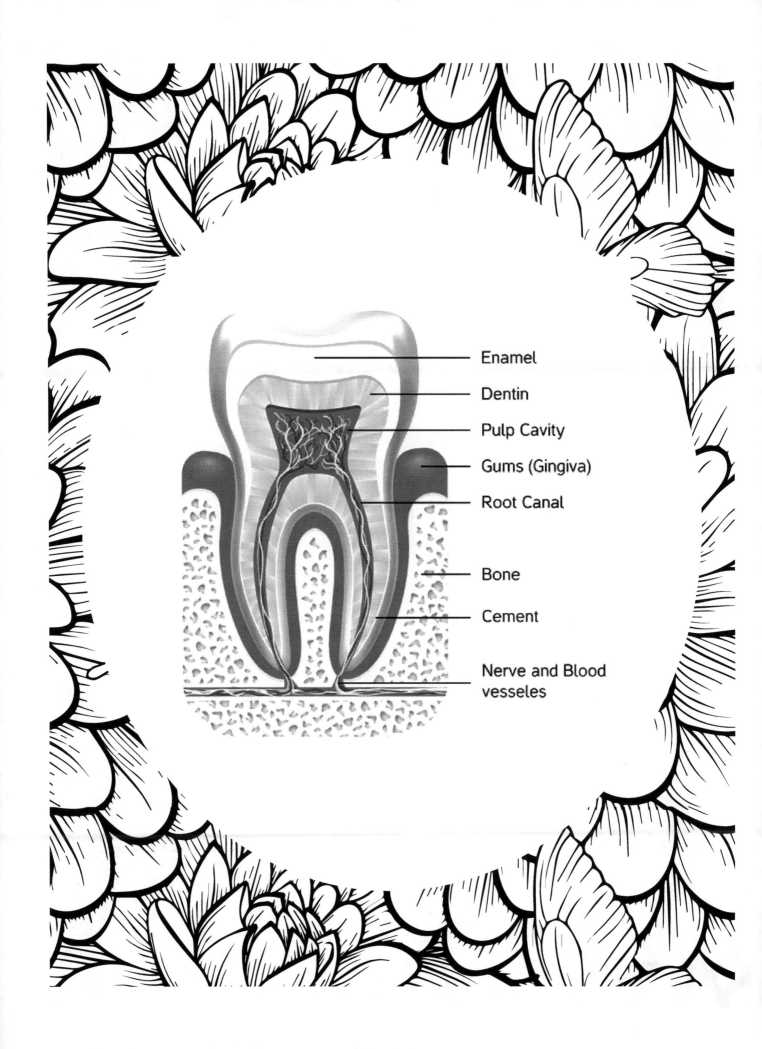

Enamel

Dentin

Pulp Cavity

Gums (Gingiva)

Root Canal

Bone

Cement

Nerve and Blood
vesseles

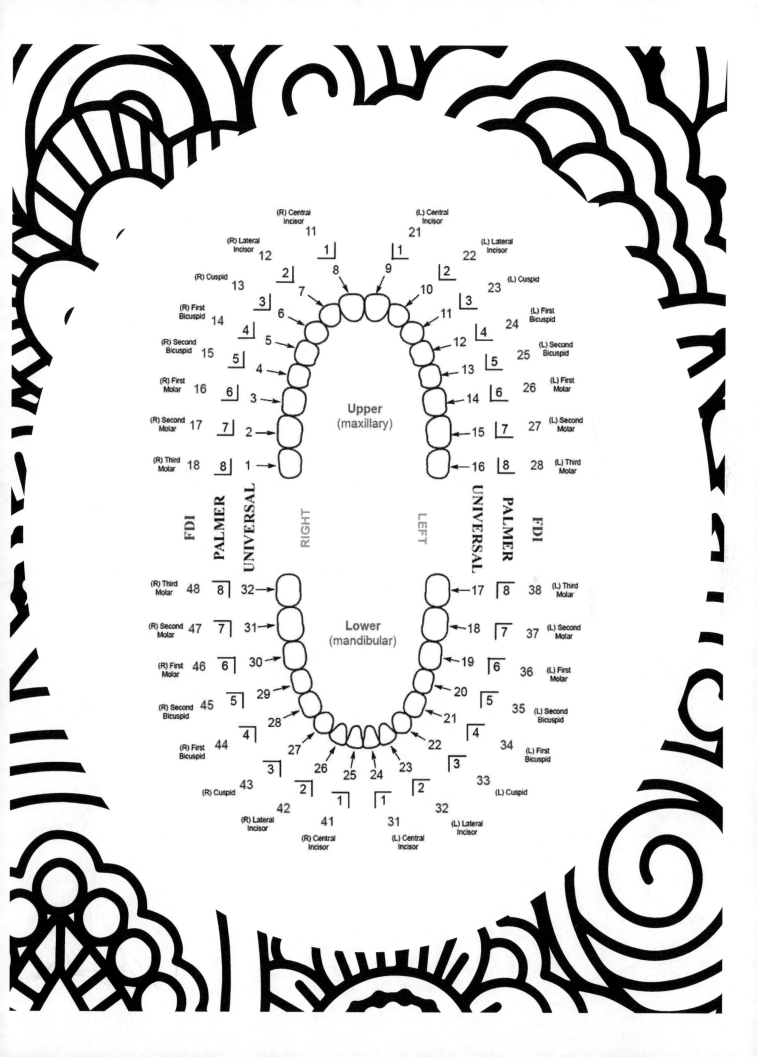

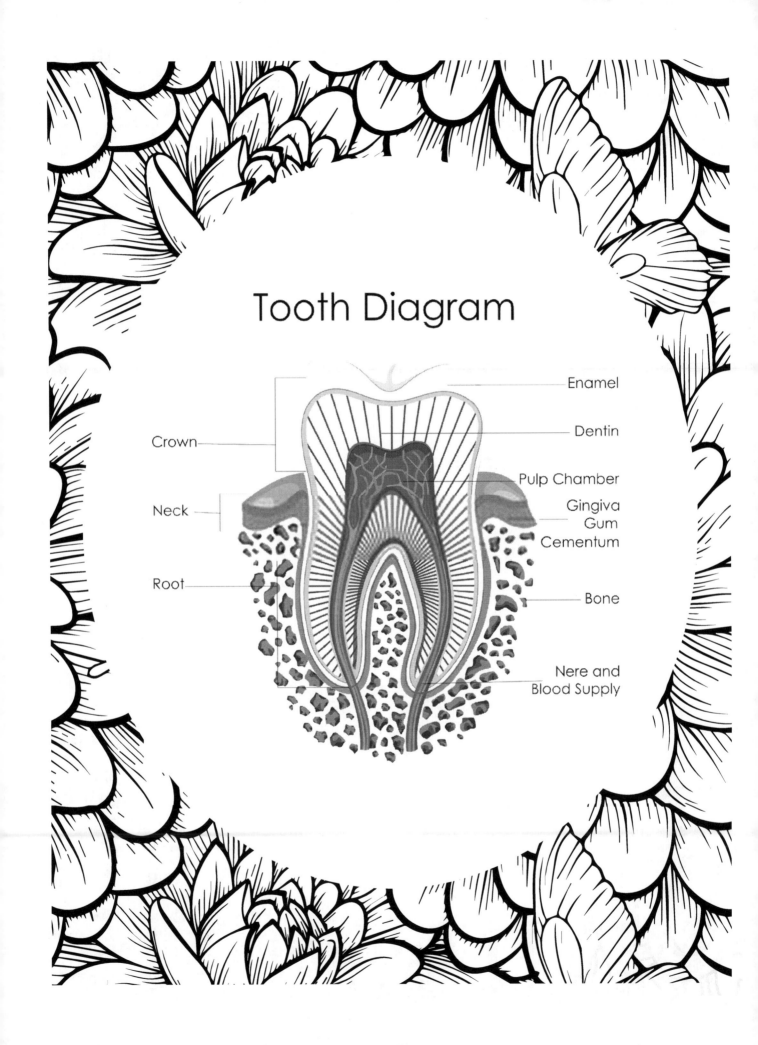

Tooth Diagram

Enamel

Dentin

Crown

Pulp Chamber

Neck

Gingiva
Gum
Cementum

Root

Bone

Nere and
Blood Supply

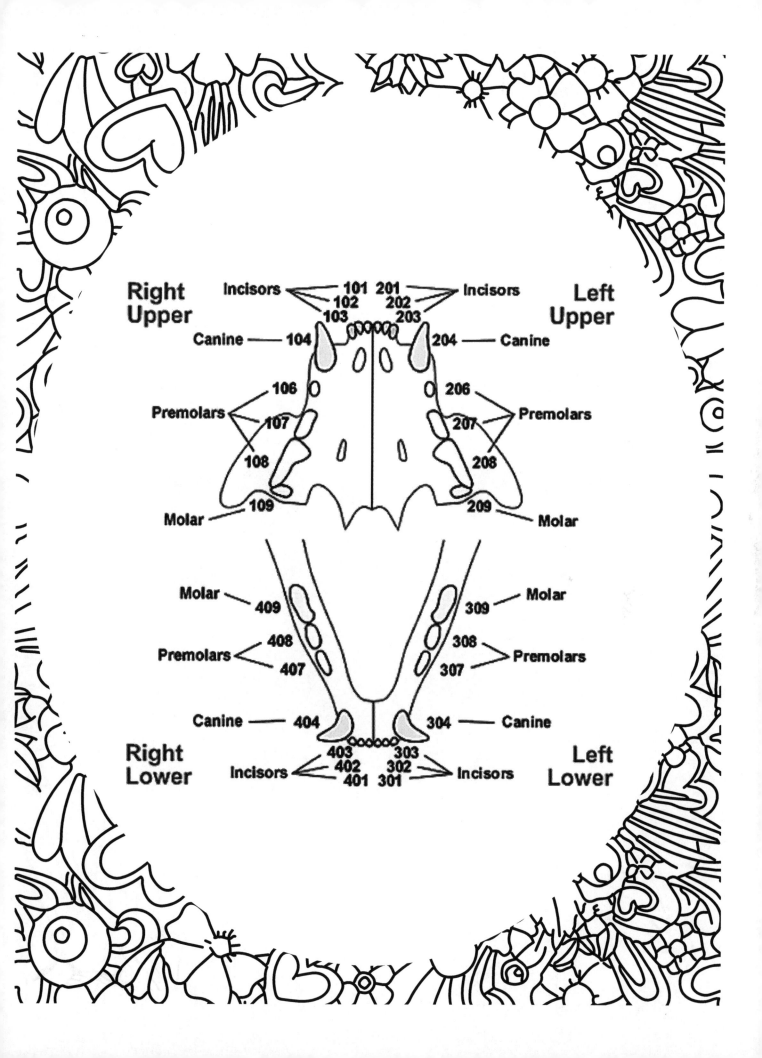

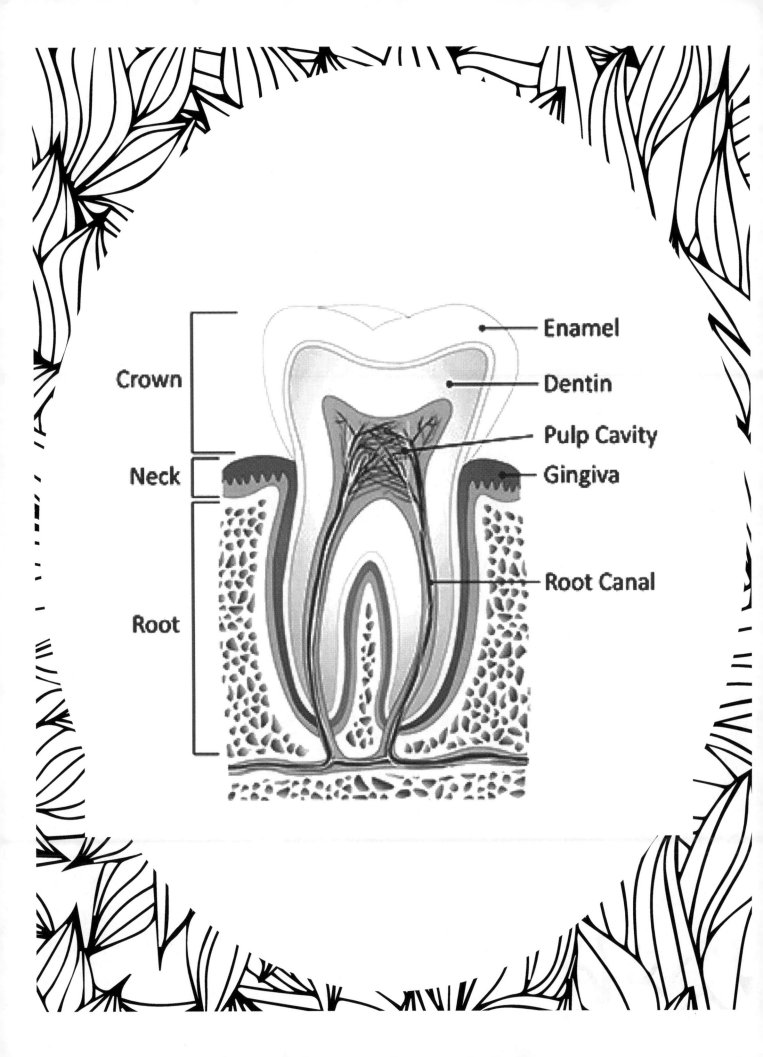

Crown

Neck

Root

Enamel

Dentin

Pulp Cavity

Gingiva

Root Canal

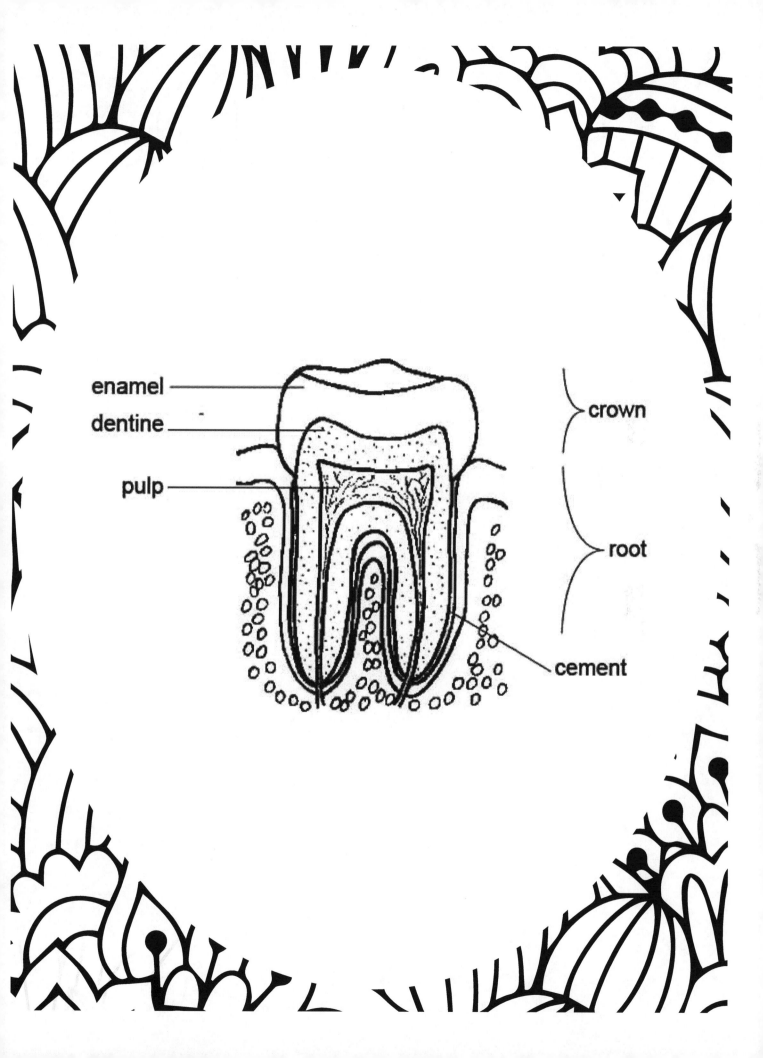

enamel

dentine

pulp

crown

root

cement

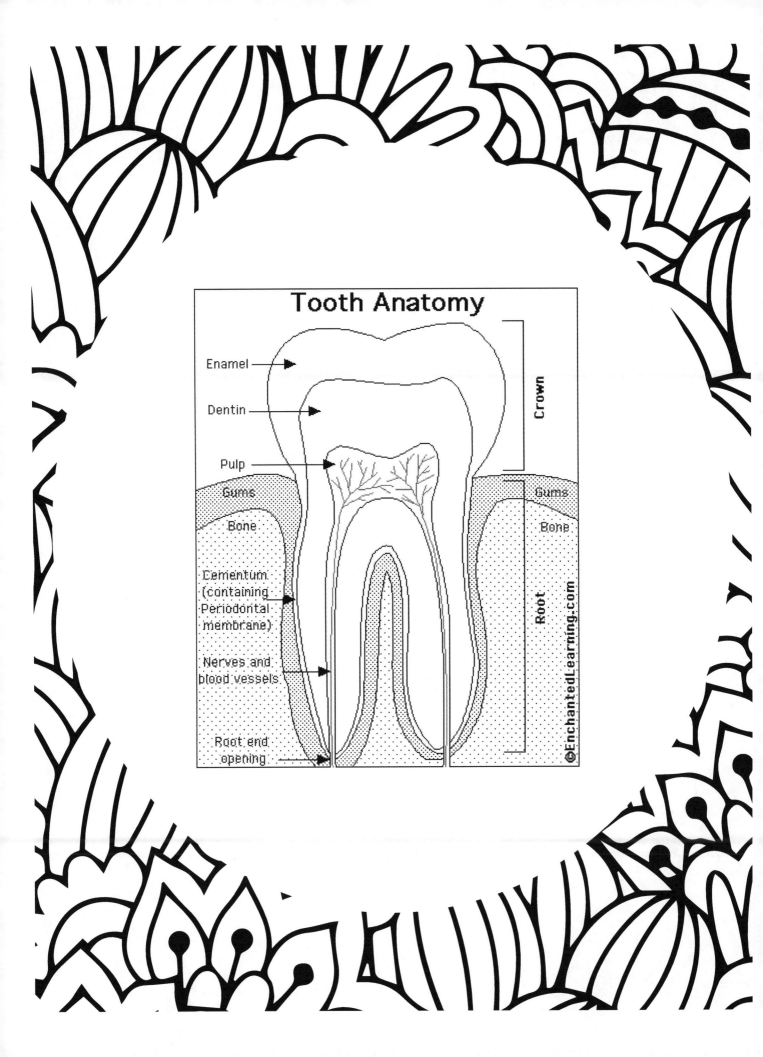

Tooth Anatomy

Enamel

Dentin

Pulp

Gums

Bone

Cementum
(containing
Periodontal
membrane)

Nerves and
blood vessels

Root end
opening

Crown

Gums

Bone

Root

©EnchantedLearning.com

40814113R00028